482

£3

used

THE FAMILY
AND THE HANDICAPPED CHILD

THE FAMILY
AND THE
HANDICAPPED CHILD

A Study of Cerebral Palsied Children in their Homes

SHEILA HEWETT

WITH

JOHN AND ELIZABETH NEWSON

London

GEORGE ALLEN AND UNWIN LTD

RUSKIN HOUSE, MUSEUM STREET

First Published in 1970
Second Impression 1972

© *George Allen and Unwin Ltd 1970*

ISBN 0 04 618012 5

REPRODUCED AND PRINTED IN GREAT BRITAIN BY
REDWOOD PRESS LIMITED, TROWBRIDGE & LONDON

ACKNOWLEDGMENTS

We would like to express our gratitude for the help we received, in the early stages of this study, from Professor Jack Tizard, Lady Jessie Francis-Williams, Dr. Agatha Bowley and Dr. M. L. Kellmer-Pringle, all of whom willingly shared with us their expertise and experience in child development and research.

We are also indebted to the staff of the Spastics Society Family Help Unit in Nottingham, not only for making it possible for us to obtain our sample but also for welcoming us to the Unit at all times, so that we could learn at first hand something about cerebral palsied children.

Our thanks also to Jean Crossland for her assistance with the field work and particularly for her secretarial services.

This study would not have been possible without the financial support of the Spastics Society, and we would particularly like to thank the Society's director, Mr. James Loring, for his interest. We must emphasise, however, that any opinions expressed in this book are entirely our own and are not necessarily shared by the Society.

Finally, to the mothers who so willingly gave us their time and the benefit of their experience, we offer our warmest thanks. Much of the content of this volume is in their words and it is to them and to their children that we dedicate our book.

CONTENTS

TABLES

INTRODUCTION

This book is a report of a research project which was designed to do three things: first, to discover what practical problems face mothers who bring up handicapped children in their own homes; second, to find out from the mothers themselves how well the various social services which are intended to help them and their children work in practice; and third, to attempt an objective comparison between the family lives of normal children and handicapped children. This last aim has been achieved by using the now extensive information about the upbringing of normal children obtained from Nottingham mothers by John and Elizabeth Newson (Newson, J. and E., 1963 and 1968), but it is important to remember two things about the comparative data. First, the normal child studies were not specifically designed to be used as part of a study concerned with handicapped children. Second, we do not claim that the use of such a sample of normal children for comparative purposes is equivalent to the use of a matched control group in an experimental situation. However, before one can claim with any justice that a group of people is behaving in an abnormal manner, it is necessary to know how a similar group behaves in similar circumstances. The only differences between the two groups compared in this book are (a) that one consists entirely of mothers of normal children and the other consists entirely of mothers who have at least one handicapped child (although, of course, the majority of them have normal children too), (b) that the children in the normal sample were all the same age at the time of interview and the children in the handicapped sample were not, and (c) the normal children all lived in the same city, the handicapped children did not. In many other respects the samples were sufficiently alike for comparison to be meaningful and to eliminate guesses and assumptions about the lives of ordinary children.

There is no shortage of literature and comment about the problems which can beset the handicapped child and his family, most of it discouraging in that discussion usually centres around the catastrophes that can occur in such families but not much is said about the families who meet the crisis of handicap, as they meet other crises, with resilience and common sense. As with the studies of normal child rearing, it is not the purpose of this book to give advice to parents on how to bring up their handicapped children. Often using the mothers' own words, we only present the picture given by the parents themselves of how they actually learn to live with a handicapped child. It is important for everyone to know how things seem from the mother's point of view, both those whose work it is to try to help them and mothers themselves who may be wondering how others feel and cope in similar situations. After a long and interesting interview, one such mother asked the interviewer, 'And now, will you answer a question for me?' The interviewer replied, 'Yes, of course—if I can,' and was then somewhat taken aback to be asked, 'Am I normal? Do others feel the way I do?' It is hoped that for her and for all mothers like her, the information in this book will be enlightening.

CHAPTER 1

ORIGIN AND CONSTITUTION OF THE SAMPLE; RESEARCH METHODS

The first problem to be solved when undertaking a project in the field of social research is that of identifying and contacting the people from whom it is necessary to obtain information—in other words, first find your sample. In the absence of any readily available comprehensive list of children known to be cerebral palsied, the Spastics Society, who commissioned the work, allowed us to use the register of children which has been compiled at the Society's Family Help Unit in Nottingham. From this source, we obtained the names and addresses of all the cerebral palsied children known to the Society who had been born in 1957 or later and were living at home with their parents in the East Midlands area—an area which included Lincolnshire, Nottinghamshire, Derbyshire, Leicestershire, Northamptonshire and Rutland. A total of 180 interviews was included in the final analysis. There is no means of knowing how many children who might have been eligible for inclusion in the sample were not on this register[1], and it must be emphasized that this work is not based on a sample randomly drawn from a known population. It is the nearest approach to a 100% sample that could be obtained. However, despite the impossibility of obtaining an ideally constituted sample, the East Midlands survey proved to be representative both in its distribution according to social class (using the Registrar General's Classification of Occupations), severity of handicap and other characteristics that one would expect to appear in a sample of children with cerebral palsy. Fortunately, there was no serious distortion of the sample through losses caused by mothers' refusal to be interviewed or by failure to make contact but, sadly, we have to

---

[1] Except in Nottingham itself—Nottingham City Health Department checked our list of children known to have cerebral palsy against their own and found only one discrepancy.

report that some children died during the period that interviews were taking place, who would otherwise have been included. A detailed account of this sample and a description of the methods used to collect and analyse the data follows.

The East Midlands sample

When the project was first planned, it had been hoped that it would be possible to contact and interview 200 mothers of children aged 7 years and under. In practice it was not possible, within the time limit set, to complete more than 180 interviews that could be included in the final analysis. This was because we had originally thought that all interviewing could be restricted to within a 30-mile radius of Nottingham, and coverage of the much greater distances that proved to be necessary was very time-consuming; and also because some interviews were completed with mothers of children who had in fact gone away to boarding school or other residential institutions. Only children who were still being cared for entirely by their parents or who were at boarding school from Monday morning to Friday evening were considered eligible for inclusion. It was felt that the latter group, 4 children in all, were still in the care of their parents for a large enough proportion of the year for parents to feel that they were not really 'away' as they would have been in an ordinary boarding school. Twenty-two children aged 8 were also included and one child had just had his 9th birthday. The numbers of children of each age are given in Table 1.I.

TABLE 1.I

Ages of children at time of interview

Age	1 yr.+	2 yrs.+	3 yrs.+	4 yrs.+	5 yrs.+	6 yrs.+	7 yrs.+	8 yrs.+	Total
Number	4	14	17	20	29	34	39	23*	180

*Including 1 child aged 9 yrs. 1 month.

Losses

Only one mother was unwilling to be interviewed. She told the interviewer that she could see no point in answering a lot of questions that had already been asked by other people. There were also two 'oblique' refusals, so described because although the mothers did not refuse outright to be seen, they always found the time suggested inconvenient. As they lived 30 and 60 miles from Nottingham respectively, and had each occasioned one fruitless journey, it was decided not to persist in trying to include them. These 3 mothers constituted a refusal rate of 2%. The total number of interviews lost, including refusals but excluding deaths, was 15 (8%) and with deaths included, was 24, (12%). A loss rate of 10% is to be expected in survey work and is generally considered to be tolerable, in particular when losses are well distributed and are not concentrated in any one category or age group. Details of all losses are set out in Table 1.II.

TABLE 1.II

Losses

Reason	Number
Child's death	9
Moved out of area	7
Direct refusals	1
Oblique refusals	2
Contacted but no interview because of language problems	3
Non-contacts because of mother's serious illness	2
Total	24

Demographic details of the sample

There were rather more boys than girls in the sample, 98 (54%) and 82 (46%) respectively. Fourteen of the children (8%) were members of twins. Illingworth[1] quotes evidence from various sources of similar findings in other studies of cerebral palsy.

The children were members of families with a size range from 1 to 10 children. The most usual number of children was 2 (28%). There were 31 'only' children (17%), 6% more than occurred in a sample of 700 normal 4-year-olds. This percentage remains unchanged when children under 4 are excluded. Forty-three (24%) were eldest children, 5% more than occurred in the same sample of normal 4-year-olds.[2] These differences are

[1] Illingworth, R. S. *Recent Advances in Cerebral Palsy.* J. & A. Churchill, Ltd., London, 1958.

[2] Newson, J. & E. *Four Years Old in an Urban Community.* George Allen & Unwin, London, 1968.

not large enough to be statistically significant and the majority of mothers were still young enough to be capable of having further children (80% of them were under 40 years old at the time of interview). There appeared to be no evidence that mothers of cerebrally palsied children tend to be older than those with normal children only, after allowing for the fact that 70% of the East Midlands children were 5–8 years old and would therefore tend to have more mothers in the older age ranges than would the normal 4-year-olds.

In 13 instances, the family included adults other than the parents living in the house. Only one of these was a lodger, the rest being relatives, mainly of the mother. Fifteen families included brothers or sisters older than 18 years who were still living at home.

Three of the children had been adopted and one was being fostered.

Thirty-nine mothers had a history of miscarriages, stillbirths and/or other children with physical disability. These are listed below:

1. Older child with dislocated hip.
2. Older child mentally retarded.
3. Older child with slight heart lesion and one miscarriage before birth of spastic child.
4. Older child with asthma, all 3 sibs described as 'slow' at school by their mother.
5. Older child with congenital heart disease.
6. Older child with congenital hip deformity.
7. Younger child with 'hole in heart' (Mother's description), one miscarriage.
8. Twin child of below average intelligence and ? epilepsy.
9. One older child with ? epilepsy and another described as 'slow' at school. One miscarriage before birth of spastic child.
10. Older child with poor sight. All children (3) born prematurely. One baby (born before spastic child) died at 3 days old.
11. Younger child with suspected heart condition, one baby (born after spastic child) stillborn.

In addition:

10 mothers had had 1 miscarriage.
 2 mothers had had 2 miscarriages.
 1 mother had had 3 miscarriages.
 2 mothers had had 4 miscarriages.

1 mother had had 5 miscarriages.

4 mothers had had 1 stillborn child.

1 mother had had 1 stillborn child and the twin of her spastic child had died after 1 day.

1 mother had had twins of which the spastic child had survived, the other being stillborn.

5 mothers had had babies who died within a week or in infancy— 1 of these children had a heart condition, another was blind and handicapped after being jaundiced; the latter died at 17 months.

1 mother had had 1 ectopic pregnancy.

Thus, 27 mothers (15%) had a history of miscarriages and/or stillbirths. Illingworth[1] cites a somewhat higher proportion found by Hopkins et al. who reported that 134 mothers out of 656, or 20%, had histories of miscarriages and stillbirths.[2]

Mothers were not asked for accounts of the births of their spastic children (although these often *were* given during the interview) for two reasons: first, such accounts were irrelevant to the main purpose of the study and second, even had birth histories been relevant, events remembered after a lapse of $1\frac{1}{2}$ to 8 years would have been of dubious accuracy and value.

[1] Op. cit., 1958.

[2] It is generally considered that mothers of cerebral palsied children more often have histories of miscarriages and stillbirths than do mothers who only have normal children. Professor Illingworth (op. cit.) quotes a rate, found by Denhoff and Holden, of 28% of their cases, i.e. of mothers of cerebrally palsied children. He also quotes Lilienfeld and Pasamanick, who found that such mothers had approximately a 35% greater infant loss than the normal population. There are difficulties, however, in relating the figures for cerebral palsy groups to normal populations. Figures for miscarriages are usually estimates because many must remain unknown for various reasons. What figures there are, are usually given in terms of pregnancies, not mothers, as in the 'Report of the Inter-Departmental Committee on Abortion (1939)' (London, H.M.S.O.). It may therefore be of interest to report the information obtained from mothers taking part in the Nottingham study of 700 normal children. At the 1-year-old stage of the survey, 16% of mothers reported at least one miscarriage or stillbirth. At the 4-year-old stage, the proportion had increased to 22%. It is known that one of these mothers also had a cerebral palsied child, as one would expect to happen in a random sample of 700 families. It is possible that there were others but unfortunately this is not known for certain. However, it *is* known that the mother already mentioned was the only one in the C.P. sample living in Nottingham who had also been included in the normal child study. As children known to have handicaps were deliberately excluded from the normal child study, it seems likely that the incidence of 22% relates to a sample of mothers the majority of whom have only normal children. If this is so, the significance of, for example, a 20% rate among mothers all of whom are known to have a cerebral palsied child, is called in question. It is not, however, intended to suggest that a history of repeated miscarriages and/or stillbirths is of no significance in this context.

About three-quarters of all the mothers were not in paid employment. Of the remaining 46, 35 were able to work part-time outside the home, 8 worked part-time at home and 1 worked full-time at home as a Local Authority foster-mother. Two mothers were working full-time outside the home; one of these was not married and worked in a factory while the maternal grandmother cared for her child, the other was the proprietress of a shop with living accommodation attached, so that she was only technically away from home when working.

These figures are compared in the table below (Table 1.III) with the numbers of mothers who were out at work in the Newsons' sample (op. cit.).

TABLE 1.III

| | Working mothers | | |
	Normal 4-year-olds (Nottingham)	Normal[1] 7-year-olds (Nottingham)	East Midlands C.P. sample[2]
	N=700	N=700	N=180
Not working	72%	56%	74%
Part-time at home	4%	6%	4%
Full-time at home	1%	—	1%
Part-time out	19%	33%	20%
Full-time out	4%	5%	1%
	100%	100%	100%

[1] The report of the 7-year-old stage of the normal child survey, from which these figures are taken, is not yet published.

[2] The abbreviation 'C.P.' is for cerebral palsied, a term which is a little more precise than the more commonly used 'spastic'. The meaning and use of these terms are discussed in Chapter 2, pp. 30–38 and in the glossary (Appendix II).

The fathers of the children were in the main in the kinds of employment that did not necessitate their staying away from home—only 1 of them was normally away during the week and 2 were often away for 3 to 5 days per week. Nine fathers had to spend nights away from home at irregular intervals. Two mothers were widows, 1 was not married, 4 were separated or divorced, but 1 of this last group was living with a man who was in most respects acting as a father to her child.

Social class distribution

The Registrar General's classification of occupations (1960) with two modifications, was used to classify families according to social class. These modifications were the same as those used in the studies of normal children.[1] Classes I and II were combined, and in 8 cases the mother's former occupation and/or training were considered to have placed the family higher in the Registrar General's scale. The East Midlands C.P. sample closely approximates to a random sample of normal 4-year-olds. Table 1.IV below compares the East Midlands Spastics sample with a simple random sample, the figures having been taken from 'Four Years Old in an Urban Community', although the actual sample of four-year-olds used for the Newsons' survey was class stratified.[2]

TABLE 1.IV

	East-Midlands C.P. sample	Simple random sample of Nottingham 4-year-olds
Class I and II	13%	14%
Class III w.c.	10%	13%
Class III man.	51%	50%
Class IV	17%	15%
Class V	9%	8%
	100%	100%
	N=180	N=500

Research methods

The project was designed to follow the precedents laid down in the course of the first two stages of the longitudinal study of the upbringing of normal children in Nottingham. The East Midlands mothers were approached by letter in the first instance and asked to give their help by telling us about their own experiences and problems. A day and time for seeing the mother in her own home was suggested, and unless she contacted the unit to alter this arrangement, an interviewer would duly arrive on the appointed day, armed with an interview schedule and a portable tape recorder.

[1] Newson, J. & E., op. cit., 1963 and 1968.
[2] Newson, J. & E., op. cit., 1968.

The interview schedule (see Appendix III) had to include questions designed to obtain factual information about a wide variety of events which affected both the handicapped child and other members of the family. In addition, we wanted the mothers to tell us what they thought and felt about some of the important issues that are bound to arise in any family, and others that become important only when one of the children is handicapped. Some of the questions that had been asked of the mothers of the normal children were included unaltered so that direct comparisons between the replies of the two groups of mothers could be made. A compromise had to be reached between the desire to include all the questions that could be considered useful and productive and the length of interview time that mothers could reasonably be expected to give. All mothers are very busy people and having a child who is handicapped is not likely to lessen their burdens. The form of schedule that emerged from our original cogitations was considerably modified, particularly with regard to question order, during pilot trials.[1] Most of the questions which did not concern purely factual matters were designed to allow the mothers to reply briefly or at length as they felt appropriate. Even more important, we did not want mothers to feel that there were any 'right' answers, that they were expected to answer in any particular way, or that one answer would meet with the interviewer's approval more than another. Question design alone will not ensure that this will be so. The interviewer and what she means to the mother can make an important difference (see Newson J. and E., 1963 for examples of differences between results of interviews conducted by health visitors and university personnel). 'Interviewer effect' is a well known and potentially troublesome phenomenon in social research.

For these reasons, as with the normal child studies, it was emphasized in the introductory letter that the interviewer was not connected with any organization or department other than the university and that she was herself the mother of a family. It was made clear that, although the Spastics Society had asked for the work to be undertaken, we were not agents for the society,

---

[1] Twenty interviews were carried out during the pilot stage of the project, 8 of these in Nottingham and 12 in East Suffolk. These 20 were not included in the final statistical analysis but made an important contribution to the general form of the results. The comments of some of these mothers have been used in the text.

nor were we a direct or indirect source of help from them or indeed from anyone. We were not there to give help or advice but simply to listen to what the mothers had to tell us.

The questions on the schedule had to be asked in the same way in every instance, but there were situations where extra 'probing' questions had to be asked in order to obtain the exact information required. Most of these extra questions were written in, but if interviewers thought it necessary they were at liberty to add *ad hoc* questions in addition to the required question. The use of tape recorders allowed constant reappraisal of interviewing techniques.

Tape recorders are invaluable for other reasons, too. Their use allows replies of any length to be recorded in full without any interruption in the flow of the story so that no nuances are lost. They guard against faulty recollection of detail on the part of the interviewer and they allow the interviewer to concentrate on maintaining the informal relationship that (she hopes) she has established with the mother. Only the briefest notes were made on the schedule as insurance against total loss should the recording prove unsatisfactory in any way. In every instance, the mother was asked if she had any objections to the use of the tape recorder and reasons for using it were given. In the event, no one in the East Midlands survey objected, and the machine was quickly forgotten as the mother became interested in answering the questions put to her. Most interviews lasted about two hours, but some were considerably longer.

The final problem is to organize the enormous amount of information obtained by these methods. Using categories which seemed to arise from the answers themselves, the information was coded and transferred to punched cards to facilitate the counting and sorting necessary before a statistical analysis can be made. In addition, to add substance to the bare bones of statistics, transcripts were made of many of the recorded interviews. Comments in the mothers' own words appear throughout the text, occasionally slightly edited to exclude complete irrelevances where this did not alter the sense, and with the names of doctors, hospitals and of course the children, omitted or, occasionally, in the case of children or their brothers and sisters, altered.

Results are presented as percentages, and where comparisons are made between the Nottingham sample of normal 4-year-olds and the East Midlands sample of handicapped children, the chi-squared test has been used to establish the level of significance of differences.

Before we can go on to present and discuss the results, however, some further points about the children must be clarified.

Severity of handicap

In order to make discussion of the problems which a handicapped child presents to his family meaningful, some measure of the degree to which his disability affects day-to-day living is essential. It was quickly realized that the medical diagnosis and categories recorded in the notes available at the Family Help Unit were not helpful from this point of view. For example, to read that a child has a left hemiplegia conveys no notion of the extent to which he is prevented from walking or talking, feeding or dressing himself, nor does it give any indication of the extent to which his actual mobility (regardless of ability to walk) is affected in his own home. These are things which his mother can tell us, and although she could not give an account in terms which would satisfy a physiotherapist or doctor, she can give a very useful description of what disability means in practical terms.

Questions about these aspects of the child were asked early in the interview, so that the interviewer was aware as soon as possible of the kind of situation she was investigating. This meant that she could avoid asking questions later in the interview which would be irrelevant to the child in question (and which would appear foolish to the mother) and also served to help put the mother at ease, since they were questions to which she was of necessity able to reply with confidence. (Some mothers greeted the interviewer with expressions of doubt about their ability to help, or to answer questions, and they were reassured to find that they could answer perfectly well.) A simple method of scoring was used for each set of possibilities; for example, a child walking unaided scored 0, those with varying degrees of walking ability were scored on a scale from 1–5, a score of 5 denoting that he was unable to walk at all. (Allowance was made for age here, using reasonable limits before which most children would not be expected to sit, walk, feed themselves or dress themselves.) Reference to the questionnaire[1] will further clarify this method

[1] Appendix III.

of scoring. No child could score an over all total of 0, since the first question concerns the number of limbs affected, however slightly. The highest possible score was 56. A rough guide to interpretation would be as follows: any child scoring less than 7 is very mildly handicapped, regardless of diagnosis and number of limbs involved, and any child scoring more than 42 is severely handicapped and very probably his score will include defects of vision, hearing and speech. Two extra categories were made to include those children whose motor handicap was relatively slight but who had a considerable impairment of sight or hearing, as it was thought that it would be misleading to consider such children to be mildly handicapped.

The children were also rated as to how far they could go by themselves, without help or supervision, regardless of their method of locomotion. This was termed their functional mobility, and in some children could be a good deal more extensive than their degree of handicap might suggest. In others, a mild physical handicap was offset by severe mental retardation, which limited functional mobility very considerably.

Using the handicap score as guide, it was found that there were equal numbers of very mildly handicapped and very severely handicapped children in the sample, 44 (25%) of the children falling into each of these two groups. The range of scores is given in Table 1.V.

TABLE 1.V

Handicap scores

ange	0–6	7–13	14–20	21–27	28–34	35–41	42–56	0–13 and blind	0–13 and deaf	*Total*
umber	44	33	18	12	11	18	40	1	3	180
	minimal/ mild		moderate			severe/very severe				

Mental assessment

As with physical disability, the records available were found to be of very little help in arriving at an estimate of degree of mental impairment. There was no question of our using psychological tests of intelligence—this lay outside the scope of the enquiry, and it is well known that it can be a long and complicated process with handicapped children.

Some clues as to the intelligence of the child were to be found in questions about schooling. If a child was attending a normal primary school, it was assumed that he had been considered to lie within the 'normal' range of intelligence, except when there was definite information to the contrary. If he attended a junior training centre, he was assumed to have been classified as 'unsuitable for education'. Some in 'special' schools were considered 'backward' according to mothers' reports. Some mothers reported that 'someone' had been to see the child to decide on his educability, although they were often not sure who this 'someone' was, and they had been told that the child could or could not go to normal school. Twenty-two children (12%) had been assessed by the Spastics Society or by the Spastics Centre in Cheyne Walk, Chelsea. It seemed fairly certain that 52 children had been assessed by Local Authority education departments and 26 by Local Authority health departments, but it should be remembered that mothers were by no means always certain of the identity of the local authority agencies who assessed their children, nor were they always told of the results.

Questions were also asked about the extent of the child's understanding of what was going on in the home and the amount of interest he took in his environment.

By these various means, it was possible to be reasonably certain that 25% of the children seen were known to be of normal intelligence or, in the case of young children who had not been tested and were not at school, gave every impression of being so. Forty-two per cent were known to have some impairment of intelligence, including 14 children for whom this was their most serious handicap. In the case of 58 children, it was not possible to make a judgment. Forty of these children responded to overtures and understood what was going on around them, 18 of them made little or no response and seemed to be apathetic. We classed all these children as being of 'uncertain' mental status, and where they are so referred to in the text it should be remembered that 'uncertain' here, means that *we* are uncertain how to classify them because of lack of information.

It is interesting to note that the percentages of children known to be of normal intelligence, or known to have some degree of mental impairment are very like those suggested by Eleanor

Schonell,[1] i.e. *about* 25% average and above, and *about* 50% mentally defective. This suggests that the rough estimates made may be accurate enough to assume that the sample of children seen is representative of all cerebral palsied children with regard to range of mental impairment, assuming that some of the children classed as having 'confirmed defects' may in fact be only slightly impaired, and some in the 'uncertain' category were in fact severely mentally subnormal.

Thirty-two of the 63 children with confirmed mental defects were also severely physically handicapped. Of the 14 children who were classified as being more mentally than physically handicapped, 9 had physical handicap scores in the range 0–13 (i.e. minimal to mild) and 5 in the range 14–34 (i.e. moderate).

General health

Mothers were asked whether their children were often ill, apart from their common condition of cerebral palsy, in particular, whether they suffered from respiratory, urinary and dental disorders.

Fifty-two mothers (29%) considered their children's health to be very good and 48 more (27%) reported only minor complaints such as colds and uncomplicated cases of measles, chickenpox and other childhood diseases. Some of these had had some bronchitis, but 75 had no health problems at all. Fifty-six of these healthy children were only minimally or moderately physically handicapped, too. Only 16 out of 62 severely physically handicapped children were reported as having good general health. They tended to have more trouble with their teeth than the less handicapped and rather more chest trouble, too.

Fits and convulsions

Estimates of the incidence of convulsions vary considerably. Two American studies, one by Hopkins, Price & Colton, the other by Perlstein & Barnet (p. 18 in Cruickshank, 1961) report their occurrence in 29·2% and approximately 40% respectively of children with cerebral palsy. Eric Denhoff, in the same volume, states that the incidence is between 35% and 60%. In the present study, mothers reported fits or convulsions in 46% of the children. Some of these included single, isolated instances

[1] Schonell F. Eleanor *Educating Spastic Children* Oliver & Boyd, Edinburgh 1956.

early in life, and 39 children (22%) had had no episodes of this kind for one year or longer at the date of interview. For 25 (14%) of the children (and parents), they were a rare occurrence, but in 5 instances they occurred at approximately monthly intervals, in 3 at approximately weekly intervals and in 11 instances were a daily hazard. Five of these 11 children were between 1 and 3 years old, the remainder between 6 and 8 years old. However, only one of the older children was having major episodes of this kind. For the other 5, they were minor episodes lasting a few seconds only. The experience of the 5 younger children was more varied. One had 3 or more major episodes per day. For another two of them a tolerable degree of control had been achieved with drug therapy, and the last two were in the process of having effective drug therapy worked out for them.

Children with mental handicap were more than twice as often reported as having fits or convulsions as were the children rated as of normal intelligence—49 or 63% of the children with confirmed mental handicap, as opposed to 13 or 29% of the children with unimpaired intelligence.

CHAPTER 2

'WHAT *IS* CEREBRAL PALSY?' DIFFICULTIES OF DIAGNOSIS AND EXPLANATION

Parents' questions must be met by discussion rather than dogmatic impressive statements in the early stages of diagnosis and treatment.

ROBERT WIGGLESWORTH[1]

It is rarely possible to be certain that a baby is cerebral palsied at the time of his birth. Unless he is very small, the baby with cerebral palsy will, in most instances, seem to his mother to be very much like any other new baby. If he *is* very small (under 5 lb. birth weight), he will be treated as a premature baby, regardless of whether he was a full-term baby or not, and given special care at the hospital until he is big enough to go home. Such babies, and also those whose mothers have encountered serious difficulties during pregnancy and/or !abour, will probably be under the care of a paediatrician for the first few months after birth to ensure that they have come to no harm as a result of such difficulties. The majority of babies attending out-patient clinics for observation in these circumstances will progress and develop normally, none the worse for having had a stormy passage into the world. Some will be less fortunate and sooner or later will begin to show signs that all is not well with them.

As well as these babies who are known to be 'at risk' for some reason, there are some who seem to have had a perfectly normal and easy introduction to life. There is no reason to suppose that their progress will not follow the usual course and yet gradually their mothers (or, occasionally, someone else) will begin to suspect that they are not quite like other babies. Their suspicions may be aroused in a number of ways and as their conviction

---

[1] Wigglesworth, Dr Robert. Contribution to a symposium on 'The Handicapped Child'. Reported in *The Practitioner*, No. 1150, Vol. 192, April, 1964.

grows that something is wrong they will begin to look for expert advice and to hope for reassurance. By the time that a mother is anxious enough to voice her fears that something is wrong with her baby, she needs above all else to be taken seriously. After all, she is the last person in the world to *want* an abnormal baby and so is unlikely to be exaggerating a situation which she dreads.

Some of these watchful and anxious mothers will sooner or later be told that their children are spastic or that they have cerebral palsy. Evidence from many surveys made over the last 20 years suggests that about 2 out of every 1,000 babies born alive have cerebral palsy.[1] In addition, some children who are normal at birth suffer a severe infection in their early lives— perhaps meningitis or encephalitis. Some of these children become cerebral palsied as a result of such conditions.

The use of these two terms is often not very helpful to mothers. What *is* cerebral palsy? Is it the same as being spastic? Great confusion can be the result of hearing these two terms used interchangeably and some mothers have gone away believing that their babies have two things wrong with them.

Cerebral palsy is in fact an 'umbrella' term used by the medical profession to cover a variety of conditions, including that of being spastic. The one thing that all these conditions have in common is that they are the result of something having 'gone wrong' with the brain. This 'something' may be a disease, an injury[2] or a failure to develop normally and it can happen before the baby is born, during birth or during the very early stages of the child's life. The result in all instances, no matter when or how the interference with the development or working of the brain takes place, is that the control exercised by the brain over the muscles of the body becomes faulty and in consequence, movement and use of the parts of the body which are affected become difficult or almost impossible. The physical handicap in particular cases of cerebral palsy may range from a slight lack of control of one limb to complete physical helpless-

[1] Illingworth, op. cit.

[2] It has been thought that injury here is rarely caused by the use of instruments in delivery. It is more likely to be the result of poor oxygen supply to the brain or of some kind of haemorrhage in the brain or a combination of the two. It can also include injuries sustained in accidents (e.g. road accidents) during the first 2 years of life. However, recent research in Birmingham by Dr Margaret Griffiths (mentioned by Professor J. P. M. Tizard of Hammersmith Hospital in an address to the Spastics Society, May 25, 1968) is suggestive that actual physical injury occurred in first-born twins, in 23 out of 25 pairs of twins studied.

ness. In addition, there may be impairment of hearing, sight and/or speech. Some of the children will also have fits or convulsions and some of them will be mentally retarded to a greater or lesser degree. Any degree of mental ability or disability may be associated with any degree of physical handicap and it does not necessarily follow that severe physical disability will be accompanied by severe mental disability, though this is often the case.

Already it can be seen why the early diagnosis of cerebral palsy is a difficult business. There are so many possibilities and the condition is very complex. It is even more difficult to predict the course of progress for any one cerebral palsied child, because although the original harm to the brain can never be undone, the child will grow and develop and the unharmed parts of his nervous system, which includes the brain, may find ways of compensating for the rest. In this way, probably much more slowly than is usual, the child with cerebral palsy may learn to sit up, to walk and to use his hands. However, the way in which he does these things is likely to be different from most people's and more difficult. In addition, he may always find it difficult to chew, to swallow and to control the expressions on his face. Because he finds it hard to swallow and to keep his mouth closed, he may dribble. If the muscles of his chest are under poor control, he may establish faulty patterns of breathing and suffer from chest complaints as a consequence. It may even be that he will never be able to walk or talk at all. On the other hand, he may be so slightly affected that none of these things happen.

There are six main ways in which the normal use of the muscles can be affected by cerebral palsy.[1] By far the most common of these is the spastic type of movement disorder, and this is the reason why all those suffering from cerebral palsy are popularly known as 'spastics'. Strictly speaking, only those whose muscles become abnormally stiff and resistant when an attempt is made to move them are spastic, i.e. have spastic cerebral palsy. Probably about 70% of all cerebral palsies are of this type. Quite different is the other most common kind of

[1] In the paragraphs which follow, we have deliberately avoided the use of technical and medical terms as far as possible. Those who would welcome a more technical description of cerebral palsy are referred to *Cerebral Palsy and Related Disorders* by Eric Denhoff, M.D. and Isabel Robinault, Ph.D. McGraw Hill, New York and London, 1960.

cerebral palsy, called athetosis. In this, the athetoid type, the muscles are not stiff and difficult to move. On the contrary, they are only too ready to move but not in the way in which the person intends them to. For example, the 'attempt to reach out and pick up a cup may result in movement of the whole of the person's body with all his limbs writhing in sympathy. These extra and unwanted movements are difficult or impossible to control. This kind of cerebral palsy is more difficult to detect in young babies than the spastic type and a firm diagnosis is unlikely to be made in the first few months of life. This is because all infants, even when they are perfectly normal, lack the ability to control the use of their muscles with the result that their movements are uncoordinated and without specific purpose. As the normal baby grows, however, his nervous system develops and becomes sufficiently mature for him to be able to make his limbs behave as he wants them to. In athetosis, this normal sequence of events does not take place, so that the child continues to show lack of coordination after the stage of development has passed at which this is to be expected.

Spasticity and athetosis are the main signs of cerebral palsy in the majority of cases. Ataxia, a condition in which coordination of movement and the ability to balance are disturbed, accounts for almost all the rest and a very small number suffer from tremor, rigidity or atony. Tremor means that there is rhythmic, uncontrolled and repetitive movement of muscles; rigidity means that limbs become very stiff for some time when they are extended; atony or atonic cerebral palsy means that muscles do not have enough stiffness and resistance when they are moved so that the child seems to be very floppy and limp.

It is possible for any child to suffer from more than one of these six types of disordered movement at the same time. Such children (and adults) have mixed types of cerebral palsy.

As well as the terms which describe the *kind* of movement disorders which may occur in cerebral palsy, there are others, equally daunting and confusing to the ordinary parent, which refer to the *extent* of these disorders. The first part of each of these terms refers to the number of limbs involved. The second part, '-plegia', is common to all of them and indicates partial or complete inability to move the limb,[1] Thus:

[1] See glossary for definitions of palsy, paresis and paralysis.

monoplegia—one limb affected (usually a leg)

hemiplegia—two limbs on the same side of the body; hence right hemiplegia or left hemiplegia

paraplegia—also refers to two limbs but always means that *both legs* are involved

triplegia—three limbs, usually both legs and one arm

quadriplegia[1]
tetraplegia } both terms mean that all four limbs are affected.

However, even the combined use of terms which give the type and the distribution of the movement disorder cannot give the whole story about any one individual since it gives no indication of the degree of severity of involvement. Nor does it give any information as to the presence or absence of any of the other handicaps that may accompany the motor disability—impairment of sight, hearing, speech and intellect, in varying degrees of severity. By the same token, it is impossible to describe a *typical* person with cerebral palsy. Each is different in some way from all the others and one is tempted to think that the cerebral palsied have only their differences in common. They also share some of their difficulties, however, and in order to bring these to life for readers who have never met anyone with any kind of cerebral palsy, we offer a small number of descriptions of some of the children we met during this project. Where quotation marks are used, the mother herself is describing her own child.

Girl: 4 yrs. 6 mths. Twin. Handicap score: 2—minimal.

A well-built, attractive little girl. The interviewer would have been unable to pick her out as the handicapped one in the family. Her mother said that her legs only were affected. She had been under the supervision of a pediatrician for the first year of her life and had had some physiotherapy. She sat up when she was just over a year old and walked without help when she was 2 years old. When seen by the interviewer, she was able to talk as well as most 4-year-olds, she could feed herself, dress and undress without help (except for back buttons), use the toilet without help, play with the other children on the little green in front of the houses. She had never had any fits or convulsions nor any feeding or sleeping

[1] In some cases two other terms are used which indicate the involvement of all four limbs—diplegia and double hemiplegia. Their use in the literature is somewhat confused but diplegia appears to indicate that the legs are more seriously affected than the upper limbs and double hemiplegia that the arms are more seriously affected than the legs.

problems. Her mother said that she was an exceptionally 'good' baby, crying very little and lying so still in her pram that she suspected when she was only 4 months old that there was something wrong—'she wasn't like the others'.

She had not had any kind of psychological assessment and her mother was expecting her to start school in the normal way with her twin.

Boy: 3 yrs. Handicap score: 7—mild.

A very well-built, nice-looking boy, very lively and active. His legs only are affected. When seen by the interviewer he was walking on his toes and his feet tended to cross.[1] He needed some support from walls and furniture when walking—where possible, hand rails had been put up for him. Double hand-rails had been made for him on the staircase, so that he could go up and down the stairs without help. His arms were very strong and well-developed, because until he started to walk at 2½ years, he had pulled himself along the floor using his arms far more than his legs. He still preferred this method of getting around when he wanted to move fast and in consequence rubbed out the toes of his shoes very quickly, often within a week of having them. He was able to talk normally for his age, feed himself and tell his mother sometimes when he wanted to go to the toilet. He had never had fits or convulsions. He had slept badly as a baby but no more so than his normal sister. He had not had any kind of psychological assessment but there was nothing in his behaviour to suggest that he was not of average intelligence.

Boy: 8 yrs. 4 mths. Handicap score: 15—moderate.

A pleasant-looking boy, very cheerful and eager to join in the conversation; a cast in one eye but the upper part of his body quite normal in appearance. His lower limbs seemed to be somewhat under-developed and his feet small (he was wearing long trousers). His mother said that all his limbs were affected but his legs more than his arms and hands. He could use scissors for cutting out pictures from magazines and used a typewriter. He was very mobile, getting around the house at amazing speed by bunny hops. He could walk with leg irons that reached to the thigh but these did not bend at the knee so that they prevented his playing with other children and slowed him down considerably. He could walk

[1] This tendency is described as 'scissoring' of the legs—the legs are pulled into such a position by faulty muscular action that they resemble a pair of scissors. The crossing occurs in various degrees of severity. When it is present without preventing walking entirely, the person is said to walk with a 'scissors' gait.

down the road to friends' house in his walking frame but preferred to use his wheelchair. He could get into and out of this without help and as he could also let himself into and out of the house, he was able to go and play with his friends as and when he liked. He needed quite a lot of help with dressing but could undress himself. He needed help with his clothes and with cleaning himself when he used the toilet and was still using nappies at night. He could not go up or down stairs. His mother said that 'someone from the education department' had come to assess him every year since he was 5 years old and he was having a home teacher for 2 hours every day. His mother thought he was 'a *little* below average' in intelligence. She saw his lack of schooling as his greatest handicap because it deprived him of the opportunity both to mix with children of his own age and to learn to be independent of her. She, too, never had any respite from him and found this her greatest problem, realizing that each had to depend too much on the other. She had no other children. She found the possibility that he would eventually have to go to boarding school very daunting, as they had never been parted, even for as long as the normal school day. 'I think that's the most trouble we've had, you know, mixing with people; I mean—he's sort of clung to me for years. I think that would be best, if they could get them away from their parents as soon as possible—nursery school or nurseries, that sort of thing.'

Boy: 8 yrs. 4 mths. Handicap score: 40—severe.

This boy was in his wheelchair throughout the interview. He seemed small for his age, with thin, under-developed limbs. His legs and arms were in constant motion, alternately contracting and shooting out uncontrollably. He could grasp objects but could not let go again at will. All his limbs were affected, and his mother said that he could use his feet better than his hands for grasping but he could not stand or walk. He could hold a pencil in his left hand, or an apple, and he could get the apple to his mouth and eat it. He could roll and wriggle around when placed on the floor, but could not get into a sitting position without help or sit without support. He was not able to dress or feed himself but he could drink from a cup. He was still using nappies, but could usually let his mother know in time when he wanted to have his bowels open. He tried very hard to talk and could make his parents understand sometimes what he meant. He took a great interest in the interview and made occasional comments which the interviewer was also beginning to understand by the time she left the house. As far as his mother knew, his sight and hearing were not impaired. He was not having fits. Unlike the 8-year-old boy in the last description, who had 4 different kinds of walking aid and a collapsible wheel-chair, this boy was presumably unable to benefit from walking aids but had a wheelchair, which did not fold, so that it could not be used for travelling. It had no tray and would not fit under an ordinary dining table, so that he could not use his hands to turn the pages of a book or have any toys to play with while he was in it. Fortunately, this boy was a weekly boarder at a special school so that he was presumably hampered by this inadequate chair during weekends and holidays only. The boy was under the routine super-vision of a pediatrician from birth, for various reasons until he was 5 years old, and the parents were told that he was severely mentally subnormal and nothing could be done for him. However, when he was almost 6, he had to spend a short period in temporary care in a hospital for the mentally subnormal because his mother was ill. During this time, he was seen by another doctor who was not convinced that he was mentally retarded to this extent and he arranged for the boy to go to a London hospital for investigation and then to an assessment centre, also in London. It was subse-quently decided that he could profit from education in a special school. Looking after such a child involves not only physical care, including a great deal of lifting and carrying, but also problems of communication and of interpretation of his wishes. As his mother said, when asked what she found most difficult to cope with, 'It's just that he can't do *anything* for himself. You see, you've got everything to do—you *think* for him, you're practically *being* him, really.'

Girl: 3 yrs. 8 mths. Handicap score: 49—very severe.

This little girl seemed very small for her age. All her limbs were affected. Her legs were crossed in the 'scissors' position described above, and the muscles of her left leg, in particular, appeared to be wasting. She kept her hands clenched with the thumbs folded on the palms, underneath the fingers. Her legs and arms moved from time to time but without apparent purpose. She was quite unable to sit up and felt very 'floppy' when the interviewer held her on her lap. Her back curved and her head fell forward on to her chest. Her sight and hearing had been tested but her mother was not sure whether her sight was impaired. Her hearing was 'all right' according to the doctor, because 'he hit his hand on the desk and she jumped.' She did not, however, make any response to over-tures of any kind during the interview and seemed completely apathetic and indifferent to her surroundings. Her eyes frequently rolled up and backwards so that the pupils virtually disappeared. She made no attempt to talk but cried a good deal during the interview. She was still in nappies, still completely bottle fed because she could only swallow liquids and spent the days and the nights in her pram beside the living room fire. Her parents took turns to sleep downstairs with her, because she woke regularly in the night for a feed, and her crying tended to disturb the other children in the family. She had fits occasionally while asleep but these seemed to be controlled by drugs at the time of interview. Her mother found feeding her the most difficult thing to cope with and no one had been able to help with this problem, although she has asked the health visitor, the home visitor from the Spastics Society and the physiotherapist who gave her weekly treatment. '*They*'ve asked around and they still don't know!' Her mother saw her total helplessness and inability to respond as the worst thing from the child's point of view—'It's not being able to do anything for herself—I mean, she won't even play with a toy. If I could just see her play with one toy, it would be something.' Her mother had been given no hope that she would ever improve and was beginning to think that she could be better cared for away from home, although she had opposed this idea when it was originally suggested to her.

Boy: 6 yrs. 7 mths. Handicap score: 14—moderate; but severely mentally handicapped.

A very well-built, nice looking boy. Both his legs are affected but when seen he was able to walk, without any appliances, as far as the local shops and go upstairs but not down. His gait was a little unusual and as he tired easily his mother had asked for a wheel-chair for taking him on longer walks. This was on order at the time of interview. He could not dress or undress himself, feed himself or tell his mother when he wanted to go to the toilet—he was still in nappies night and day. He had had convulsions earlier in his life but these had been controlled by drugs which he had been taking since he was 2 years old. He had had a squint which had been corrected and his hearing was impaired. He did not have a hearing aid. He had no speech—'We just get the noises. That's what makes it so difficult—when he starts to cry he's so upset. It's always more guesswork, as it is with a new baby, really.' To the interviewer, the most striking thing about this boy was his un-ceasing aimless activity. Throughout the interview, he was walking or running about the room, humming tunelessly or squeaking loudly. Sometimes he would bang his head against a wall in the course of his wandering. Then his mother would turn him round and set him on a new course, remarking that he would otherwise go on banging his head because he did not understand that he could not get through the obstacle. He did not once meddle with ornaments, electric plugs or attempt to open the door during the interview, and the interviewer got the impression that this was because he was not sufficiently interested in anything to be prompted to do so. He rarely looked directly at a person even when spoken to. When asked what she found most difficult to cope with, his mother said, 'I think it's dreadful to see a young child not doing the same as the other children that you know are the same age—going off to school and you're still stuck with yours here— you know. About what's going to happen to him when you're not there, who will look after him when you can't look after him— will they be kind to him. You know, the usual type of thing. The fact that he can't do anything for himself; he's so completely dependent on you . . . he could starve at the side of food.' His mother had recently asked if she could see another pediatrician for a second opinion. This second doctor had advised her to arrange for him to be cared for in an institution. He suggested that she agree to having his name put on a waiting list as it would be some years before a place could be found for him. Meanwhile she was hoping that he would be able to attend a junior training centre in the near future.

This small selection of differing degrees and kinds of handicap may help to indicate the complexity of the conditions that share the common designation of cerebral palsy. One really needs to *see* cerebral palsied children to understand how their disordered movements affect their general appearance, because actual deformities of limbs often do not become obvious until later in life, when prolonged lack of use has resulted in permanent contractures. When children as young as those in the East Midlands sample are relaxed and lying or sitting at rest, their handicaps could remain unnoticed by the casual observer, if it were not for the fact that they are in wheelchairs or in prams and push chairs after the age when this is to be expected.

The presentation of these complicated facts to worried parents in terms which they will be able to understand, calls for considerable tact and ingenuity on the part of the doctors. All parents are different and all children are different. We asked the mothers in the East Midlands what their experiences had been, and invited their opinions on how this difficult and painful task can best be tackled.

To go back to the point made earlier, we discovered that 90 % of all the mothers we talked to already thought that something was wrong with their babies before they were told that they were spastic. In some cases, they had taken the children to doctors, but the doctors were unwilling or unable to commit themselves to a definite diagnosis, although they did believe that something was wrong. In other cases, mothers were unable to convince anyone that there was really anything wrong with their babies and this added greatly to their anxiety. Here are some examples of their stories, in their own words:

Girl: 3 yrs.

> I wasn't happy about her because I used to put her on the floor and she didn't do *anything*. She just lay there and I thought, 'Well, that's not right'. And I asked our doctor and I asked Dr —— and they all said there's nothing wrong with her. But I wasn't at all happy. I'd put her down and she wouldn't move at all. And then someone said 'Perhaps she's a lazy baby'—somebody else said, 'Oh, you can't possibly *have* a lazy baby'—but if you go to doctors and they keep telling you nothing is wrong, what *are* you to do?

Boy: 5 yrs.

> When he was a year, I kept going to the doctor and I kept saying 'I'm sure there's something wrong with him', because he wasn't walking or sitting up and he was nearly a year old. And the doctor says 'You don't judge babies by other babies'. Well, I know that, but it was just worrying so I went to the clinic and spoke to the doctor there and *he* says 'Well, we can't go over your own doctor's head, but we can send you to see (the paediatrician) at our other clinic.' And that's how I got there.

Boy: 8 yrs.

> Well, I told them at the clinic and they wouldn't believe me. When he was about 4 or 5 months old—give him a rattle or anything like that, a baby will hold it and *he* wouldn't, he just—put it into his hand, his hand would just open and he'd drop it. And they just called me stupid, at the clinic. He *looked* a very healthy child, by the look of him you wouldn't think there was anything wrong with him at all. I knew as early as 4 months old, he wasn't holding things—I thought 'Well, he should be holding things'. They sort of laughed—you know. And then when he would't sit up they said—I think I told them when he was about 8 or 9 months old—and they said, 'Oh, he's a big baby, he'll sit up'. Then when he wouldn't walk, they wouldn't do anything until he was 19 months old, about him not walking . . . The clinic just ignored me, as much as to say, 'You don't know anything about it'.
>
> (Mother had been a nursery nurse)

Girl: 7 yrs.

She was about 8 months old and she wasn't sitting up and she kept this little hand clenched. The doctor said she was just lazy, because she wasn't sitting up properly. He said, 'Oh, she's a fat baby, she's lazy, she's not, you know, she's not bothered.' She just used to lay there, she didn't make any attempt to do anything, really.

Boy: 18 mths. (Pilot study)

Well, I've had Joycie, she were premature and I had ever such a lot of trouble with her, but she weren't like this. She couldn't walk till she were nearly three and she couldn't sit up at all till she was two, but I *did* know that there were something *different* in him—I mean, Joycie did use to take notice of you and she *started* to sit up and she always fed herself. I rang for the doctor one day—I was breaking my heart when he came. So he said, 'What's the trouble?' and I told him 'There's something wrong, what it is I couldn't tell you. But I'm not satisfied with him. He doesn't take that much notice, doesn't try to sit up, he takes no interest in what's going on around him'—and that was at eight months. So he said 'Now, look here, Mrs ——, what can you expect? He was just over 2 lbs. born, he was premature, and you've done very well with him to pull him through the way you have. But anyway', he says, 'there's nothing wrong.' I said 'Well, he's always crying'—I just *knew* he wasn't what he ought to be.

Girl: 6 yrs.

Well, I wasn't really told at all, I just found out for myself. When a baby is born, like, the first thing they do is nestle to your breast, isn't it? Well, she never did that—she wouldn't have a bottle and she wouldn't have a dummy and I knew there was something wrong from then, like.

These children were of different ages, only one of them being under two years old at the time of interview and this suggests the possibility that the greater awareness of the nature of cerebral palsy in recent years would mean that mothers of children under two would have had somewhat different experiences. Out of 21 mothers in the sample whose children were born in 1963 and 1964, only 6 reported that they found it difficult to convince anyone that there was anything wrong with them.

However, some doctors still seemed to be reluctant to put a name to the children's condition. Only 7 of these 21 mothers were told what was wrong before the children were one year old, 3 of these before they were three months old. But still 3 mothers of these 21 younger children had found out *by chance* what was wrong—one had overheard the word spastic when the consultant was talking to a colleague and the other 2 had read it on an appointment card and a referral note respectively.

It is probably difficult for the doctor to decide how and when to tell the mother that her child has a condition for which he can offer no cure. But when parents are already suspicious and anxious, it is mistaken kindness to keep them in suspense any longer. We asked mothers whether they would prefer to be told when the doctor himself suspects something is wrong (although he may not be sure what it is), or whether they would rather he waited until he could give them a definite diagnosis. The majority of them (70%) felt that doctors should tell parents as soon as they suspect that something is wrong, even though they cannot be sure exactly what it is. There is a strong feeling that mothers have a right to information about their children, particularly as they have the duty of caring for them. What is quite clear is that in most cases one plain, bald statement of the facts, however simply they may have been put, will not be enough. Mothers themselves made the point that on being told initially, they were too upset to take in much of the explanation. Some of them suggested that the person with whom to discuss the diagnosis is the general practitioner, who could be informed of the diagnosis by the consultant, and could then visit the parents to answer any queries or doubts they might have. Whatever the merits or demerits of this approach might be, it is clear that someone should be available to give repeated explanations. The need is for discussion, as the quotation at the head of this chapter suggests, but it may be unrealistic to wait for questions from the parents before initiating such discussion. Mothers feel at a disadvantage when they are dealing with professional people, and even if given time to do so, may be too diffident to ask the questions that have been troubling them between visits to the consultant. The feelings of many mothers were expressed by the one who said: 'They don't sit and explain anything—sometimes you feel sort of inadequate—you can't talk the same way as they can. They treat you as though, if they told you, you

wouldn't understand; but I think every mother ought to know.'
(Boy: 3 yrs.).

Another, who was eventually offered the chance to ask questions that she had always wanted, found herself tongue-tied when the time came, as she ruefully explained to the interviewer:

Girl: 8 yrs.

> I went up to see Dr —— just before she went into . . . (a hospital for short-term care) and I was on about the evasiveness of everyone concerned and—I think there were four of them in the room at once—and he said, 'Well, go ahead and ask your questions.' I was struck dumb—I didn't know what to say! (Laughs) I never felt such a fool in my life. 'I don't know what to ask you—for years I've thought well, it's no use asking people and if you have asked them you've got no answers'. And I think I did ask them how bad she was and he turned round so matter of fact and said, 'Well, from what we know of her we think she'll progress to about 14'. As I say, it shook me rigid—I went home in tears. I'd never been told that before. (Laughs) I was a fool.

Just over half of the mothers we saw said that they had not had their children's condition explained to them. Some of these mothers had found out a great deal themselves, but some were quite happy not to know too much, partly because they were frightened of what they might hear but also because they felt that merely *knowing* would not help the situation.

Although about half the mothers had not had the kind of discussion that is thought to be desirable, this did not necessarily mean that they felt dissatisfied with the way in which they had been told the diagnosis. Of the 150 who had been told by someone (not necessarily the consultant), a large number (70%) were satisfied with the way the news had been given to them. Often the fact that they had been told at all, however bluntly, was what counted, and among those who were not satisfied were some who were eventually told by consultants only after they had felt for some time that something was being kept from them. Although the majority view is that parents should be told of the doctor's suspicions, there are other ways of looking at this problem. Mothers gave very thoughtful replies to this question—it is obviously something which matters a great deal to most of them. Some examples of the variety of their opinions are given below.

Girl: 7 yrs.

I think he should tell you of his fears. After all, if he *thinks*, then there must be something there to make him think. You might wait a year for confirmation, dependent on the child, specially one that's not too badly handicapped.

Boy: 6 yrs.

I think it's a good idea to wait because parents get used to it, they grow accustomed to it whereas the shock of it might upset them so much it could have a lasting effect, whereas when you get used to it you sort of—I don't know—I think it's a good idea to tell them gradually, keep them guessing a while, because nobody really knows exactly. I mean, it might turn out to be perfectly all right.

Girl: 3 yrs. (Pilot study)

Parents are so different and for myself, I think I'd rather have known, because I was never at ease and I couldn't make out why she didn't *do* more, and every time you asked you never got a definite answer. But I think with some parents it would be better to wait until it was definite. I think it's very hard, I think it's something the doctor possibly has to decide—he must see a lot of people—he must be able to sum them up to a degree, mustn't he?

Boy: 4 yrs.

Well, I think a mother should be told straight away, you see, but . . . there's a way of telling people. I think if people *are* going to be told, the husband and the wife together should be told. It should be explained to them more kindly than the way I was told. I mean, I was completely alone with the specialist and he wasn't a very nice man, either. I suppose he may have thought he was being quite kind—I don't know. I think he should tell them even if he had the slightest suspicion of anything wrong—even if there isn't —it's either a relief if you're told there *is* nothing wrong or you half expect it if there *is* something wrong.

Girl: 6 yrs.

Well, I do think it is best to be told as soon as possible, but I think it's something you've got to accept, you've got to learn to accept; personally, I'd rather be told all the facts and know exactly what's going on, than have a lot of whitewashing. If there is no hope, I'd rather be told. I think as regards telling a person, I think once all the tests have been done, to eliminate any sort of medical thing apart from either spasticity or mental handicap, I think then that both parents should be told together, all the facts that they could understand. I think they should be told quite plainly and as soon as possible.

Boy: 5 yrs.

There isn't a right moment. Well, I've spoken to a lot of different people about this and I haven't got any proper feelings myself, you know. I think I wouldn't have liked to have known straight away about him when he was born, when he was a baby. I think I would have been frightened of him when he was a little baby, spoilt him and coddled him too much, I think, and not let him be normal at all.

Boy: 6 yrs.

We never have been told, really . . . well, we've known, you know, it's gradually dawned on us. I don't think I could have stood being told.

Lack of time probably accounts to some extent for the absence of discussions. Mothers' estimates of time spent with the consultant on routine visits rarely exceeded 10 minutes, and some thought it was less. The intervals between visits varied from 1 month to 12 months, 6 months being the most usual—30% of the whole sample gave this as the interval between attendances at the time of interview. Children who are being watched carefully because they were premature or have had difficulties at birth, are often seen as frequently as once per month during the first few months of their lives, which can be very difficult for their mothers, particularly when they have other young children. However, this degree of contact with the specialists is soon reduced to 3 or 6 monthly routine visits as the child gets older, and eventually 12 months may elapse between visits. Referring only to these regular, routine visits to the consultant in charge of the case and excluding visits made to other specialists such as orthopaedic surgeons, ear, nose and throat specialists and others, we asked mothers how helpful they had found such visits. We found that when mothers always saw the same doctor, almost equal numbers of them were satisfied or non-commital (54 mothers) as were dissatisfied (50 mothers) while 2 out of 3 mothers who saw different doctors were dissatisfied. Of this last group (28 mothers), the most common source of dissatisfaction was that a large proportion of the already short consultation time had to be spent in putting the doctor in the picture, not in receiving advice themselves. Mothers in the other group complained frequently that the short time spent with the consultant was a poor exchange for the length of time spent waiting to see him. Others felt that no useful purpose was served by the visits from their point of view, as they were not told anything when they got there but that they might be helpful for the doctors.

Boy: 7 yrs.

They're so busy they can't really give the time. It's just a waste of time to be got in—'Oh, yes. Well, you're going on all right'— pick up your clothes and pass on. Sometimes I feel it's a bit half-hearted. It's a matter of routine, going there.

Boy: 8 yrs.

I took him to see Mr M. last October and all he said—I was in there about 2 minutes, that's all—he just took his shoes and socks off and said 'Bring him back in another 12 months'. Well, that's all you get to know and to me that's an afternoon just wasted. If they *tell* you and explain things to you, that would be different but they won't.

Girl: 7 yrs.

Well, it doesn't help *me*—they just take her height and weight, ask me how she's been, like, but they never discuss anything, you know.

Boy: 6 yrs.

Well, to me they're not, really. But whether they are to them or not, I don't know. They just have a look at him.

When mothers are dissatisfied, they often comment on the lack of discussion, not lack of treatment—they are well aware that there is not likely to be anything positive to help the children, apart from physiotherapy or other therapy. Similarly, when mothers say that visits are helpful, it is usually because they regard them as opportunities to talk things over.

Girl: 7 yrs.

Very helpful. Because, as I say, that is the only time that I *can* talk to somebody—our own doctor is no good, so therefore I look forward to it, really.

Boy: 6 yrs.

> I think when you've had a talk to someone who knows about these things you feel more relieved—I know I do, anyway.

These mothers have been fortunate in that they have been able to see the consultant as an ally, but the first of the two mothers quoted above also said when discussing this topic:

> I'm not frightened of him, not in any way. I speak my mind, I've learned that, all these years of struggling with her and seeing different doctors—you know—and having to fight for the child all the time, which you *do* have to do. Because she can't fight for herself, therefore you have to do it.

This was not the only reference to the feeling that parents have to fight for their children, the feeling that doctors (and other professional people) are opponents rather than allies, to be approached with a mixture of caution and militance rather than confidence.

The real problem seems to be diffidence on the part of both mothers and doctors about initiating discussion. The last word on the subject goes to a mother who sums up her predicament like this:

Girl: 2 yrs.

> The first thing I knew, it was on this card. It said, 'Nature of case—Spastic'. I never dreamed she was a spastic—I mean, I'd never had owt to do with spastics. You don't take no interest until you've got one of your own, I don't think. (Interviewer: Did you say anything to the doctor after you'd read it on the card?) No; you see, I've never really *spoke* to him—I've never asked him anything. And that's another thing—you've *got* to ask, haven't you, really? But I never have. I s'pose I expect *him* to talk to me, but . . .

CHAPTER 3

PRACTICAL ASPECTS OF
DAY-TO-DAY LIVING

*The effects of a disability must always be judged in
relation to the present and future circumstances of the
person concerned.*

JOHN D. KERSHAW[1]

The degree to which a disability becomes a handicap depends to
a certain extent on the surroundings of the person who is
disabled. Being unable to walk upstairs, for example, might not
be a serious restriction on a child living in an African village
where the huts were all on ground level, but it would be a problem to a child living in a community which builds its houses on
stilts, as they do in parts of New Guinea. In the same way, the
difficulty of caring for handicapped children in our own society
can be increased by unsuitable housing and lack of appropriate
equipment or aids to overcome the problems.

In some areas of Great Britain the housing shortage is acute,
and this shortage is inevitably reflected in surveys of the needs
of handicapped children.[2] The situation in the East Midlands
area is not so acute. None of the cities in the area covered by
this survey[3] has the same population problem as London,
which is a magnet for labour of all kinds, nor have they the
housing situation that Glasgow faces with a high proportion of
tenement accommodation. Council housing that affords a good
standard of amenities forms a considerable proportion of the
housing available in Nottingham, for example. This is mostly
situated on large estates and consists of two-storey houses with
gardens. Multi-storey building has become an important part of
the city's housing programme only within the last ten years.

[1] Kershaw, John D.: *Handicapped Children*, London, Heinemann, 1966.
[2] As in the Glasgow survey, reported in the Carnegie United Kingdom Trust
Report, 1964.
[3] See Chapter 1.

About 39 % of all the housing in the city has been purpose-built by the corporation. Some of the oldest properties have been purchased by them under slum clearance schemes, but some of the 19th century terraced housing in Nottingham and other Midland towns is well built and still serviceable. It lacks the amenities, of course, that are provided as a matter of course in modern housing, unless these have been added under improvement schemes.

The East Midlands mothers lived in widely differing areas, ranging from the large cities to isolated villages in rural areas, in every type of housing. Thirty-seven had houses with outside toilets only (6 of them without water), but these were not shared by more than one family. Most mothers did not say that an outside toilet was an inconvenience, either when we asked the general question, 'Is there anything about the house you find inconvenient?', or when we asked specifically about this as an item in our check-list of amenities. This is a small but interesting instance of a finding that was contrary to what might have been expected by people who consider an inside toilet a necessity, particularly where there is a handicapped child. There are two things to remember, which go some way to explain it in the present context. The first is, that where the handicapped child was incontinent and the mother had resigned herself to this, giving up all attempts at toilet training, the location of the toilet was not of any greater significance than for any family. The second point is, that mothers who had been brought up with outside toilets were so used to this that they had never thought of it as being particularly inconvenient. This is not to say that they would not have appreciated an inside toilet if they had been given the opportunity to have one.

A similar point must be made with reference to bathrooms— or their absence. Eighteen families had no bathroom but only 4 mothers mentioned this as an inconvenience. Nevertheless, it *is* more convenient to have an inside toilet and a proper bathroom with hot water on tap—the experience of some of the mothers in the normal child sample is of interest here. Those who were interviewed after they had been re-housed on a modern housing estate were asked what they liked best about their new homes in comparison with the old terraced houses they had left behind; the bathroom was cited more often than anything else. Mothers had not realized how much difference a proper bathroom could make to their lives until they actually had one.

The general question about whether mothers found anything at all that was inconvenient about their homes, was followed by a specific check on toilets, bathrooms, gardens and laundry facilities, including hot water systems and drying areas. One hundred and ten (61%) of the sample had no complaints to make. The things the remainder specifically mentioned as inconvenient are listed below (Table 3.I).

TABLE 3.I

Housing problems

Problems	Number of houses
Awkward stairs	18
Bathrooms—too cold or too small	3
No bathroom	4
Toilets—because upstairs	7
because outside	3
because not flush	5
Damp	3
Awkward steps	10
Sloping yard	4
Narrow doorways	3
Totally unsuitable	5
Complaints not specific to handicapped child only, e.g. house too small, only one living room, insufficient storage space	21

All types of housing were subject to criticism, including modern detached and semi-detached houses. A few parents who could afford to do so had acquired bungalows because of their greater suitability both for the handicapped child and for those looking after him. At the other extreme, there were the 5 families living in totally unsuitable accommodation. This included a caravan; a single rented room in an old terraced property, used for living and sleeping; two cottages in rural areas and one council-owned terraced house, scheduled for demolition. This house was in a truly deplorable condition, with the back kitchen falling away from the main part of the house, so that one could look up into the bedroom above through the gap. Six families had been given priority on local authority housing waiting lists, and one more was hoping to be re-housed in the same way in the near future.

Sometimes quite a small alteration would have made a big difference to the child's ability to get around the house without help. One mother, for example, felt that a hand-rail each side of the stairs, at a height which the child could reach, would be a great help to her child, but the distance between them needed to be less than the actual width of the staircase. In another home this idea had been put into practice by a handyman uncle. He had made a hand-rail of metal tubing low down on the staircase wall and another up the centre of the staircase. This centre rail was on metal supports screwed to the stair treads. This enabled the 3-year-old boy to swing himself up and down stairs with great agility and enjoyment. He could do this without help from another person, thus greatly contributing to his independence. This is a very important point. The main purpose of special adaptations and gadgets is that the handicapped child should achieve the greatest measure of independence that is practicable within the limitations set by his disabilities. A mother in the pilot sample had met opposition to the idea of providing rails in the toilet that would enable her 6-year-old son to manage to use the toilet without help. She said:

> I did bring this up with someone because I felt rather strongly about it. I have thought that one ought to be able to have things fixed up in order to make it easy for them—to make it *possible* for them, not really easy—but so they can do the normal things as normally as possible. I don't know if it was Dr ——; I wouldn't swear to it, but he said that the less special sort of equipment they have the better; try to do things in the ordinary way. I don't know whether that's very sensible always—it might mean that they're not doing it at all.

There is probably a balance to be struck between having too many aids and too few, but the important thing, surely, is to 'make it possible', as this mother says. A child can learn later to do without props which are really not essential.

Twenty-five fathers had either made alterations to their homes themselves or had had them done privately. Many of these were relatively minor, such as putting up hand-rails where necessary, making barricades for staircases and putting up extra fences in the garden. Two had added rooms on the ground floor. Five had put in toilets and/or bathrooms downstairs.

We asked whether the local authority had helped towards making alterations to homes which would help the handicapped child. We were given only five instances of such help, all in council houses. These are given here to illustrate the variety of ways in which local authorities can help: a small toilet installed; doorway enlarged and path made; a fence put up; path made and small storehouse for the wheelchair; a hand-rail on the stairs. Two more mothers were still waiting for alterations that had been promised, in one case in a privately rented house. In another two instances a visitor from the Welfare Department had called to see if any help of this kind was required but both these families were living in owner-occupied modern detached houses and needed no help.

The majority of mothers in the sample were surprised when we asked this question and seemed unaware that such service was available. Local authorities have permissive powers, under the National Assistance Act, to provide help for the handi-capped in their homes through their Health and/or Welfare Departments. The amount and kind of assistance is not speci-fically laid down in the Act, so that provision may vary from one authority to another. It is also possible that there is a breakdown in communication about this service. Parents do not ask for help because they do not know they can. They therefore make little demand on the Welfare Departments for this kind of help. This fact in its turn may lead Welfare Officers and Medical Officers of Health to believe that needs do not exist. A vicious circle is therefore set up. It would be unfor-tunate for the Welfare Departments who may be ready and willing to supply help and for the families in need, if mutual ignorance of each other's existence were the only stumbling block to meeting needs.

Turning now to the children themselves, some way has to be found which will give a picture of their lives in their own homes and the range of problems with which they confront their parents from day to day. The age range of the sample, the variety of the handicaps they suffer and the varying importance of these handicaps to the child and to the family, mean that it is difficult to generalize about the sample as a whole. Nevertheless, an overall picture of the incidence of both handicaps and prob-lems is a useful point from which to start discussing more individual aspects of handicap. Table 3.II gives a list of the kind of problem mentioned by mothers and the number of children having these problems.

TABLE 3.II

Incidence of disabilities/management problems

	No. of children	%
Unable to sit at all without support[1]	56	31
Unable to walk at all	69	38
Functional mobility nil	56	31
Functional mobility confined to one room	11	6
Unable to put on clothes without help	124	69
Unable to feed himself without help	67	37
Unable to drink from a cup/uses feeding bottle	32	18
Difficulty with chewing and/or swallowing	63	35
Doubly incontinent	67	38
Impairment of vision (known to mother)	66 (inc. 4 blind)	36
Impairment of hearing (known to mother)	15 (inc. 1 severely deaf)	8
Impairment of speech: 1. slight/moderate	31	17
2. serious	21	12
3. can say 1–2 words only	27	15
4. no speech	52	29
Sleeping problems: 1. getting to sleep	52	29
2. waking often during night	18	10
3. waking sometimes during night	96	53
Fits/convulsions	44	24

[1] It follows that if children cannot sit they cannot stand or walk either.

When considering whether a problem or disability exists for any one child, proper allowance has been made for the fact that some had not yet reached the age by which particular skills have usually been acquired by normal children. Children with the highest handicap scores would have most of the difficulties listed above.

Obviously the size of the children makes an important difference to the difficulty of caring for them. For example, the small girl of three described on page 36 is less difficult to carry and lift than the 8-year-old boy described on page 35, although her handicap score is 49 and his 40. The length and the weight of the children inevitably makes procedures like bathing, dressing and changing nappies a great deal more arduous after the age of

5 and possibly before this is they have grown normally. There were 23 children aged 5 or older who could not sit unsupported. Twelve more in this age group had some sitting balance but could not stand without support and another 13 could sit and stand but could not walk at all. Thus rather more than a quarter of the sample (48 children) presented management problems on this count alone. Thirty-six mothers said that lifting and carrying heavy children were their greatest problems.

For children such as these, various appliances and equipment are supplied by the National Health Service. There are also children who can walk but only with the aid of walking frames or calipers. These, too, are supplied by the National Health Service. Twenty-two children in the East Midlands sample (12%) had only a wheelchair, a further 29 (16%) had a wheelchair plus at least one other piece of special equipment. Thirty-five children had special adjustable indoor chairs, known as Amesbury chairs. These are usually specifically designed to fit individual children, taking into account differing needs for support and control. They can be moved around on castors or wheels and tilted backwards if necessary. Wheelchairs often have to be modified to meet individual needs, too. For example, 'wings' have to be added for children who have poor head control. Children whose legs tend to cross need a padded wooden pole or block fixed to the seat to prevent this happening.

Almost half the sample had no special equipment for the children at the time of interview. Thirty-eight mothers had made requests for various items, which had not been met—possibly in some cases because the item requested was not in fact really suitable for the child concerned. In other cases, however, the reason seemed to be that there had been some confusion about how to obtain it. We will return to this point later in this chapter.

The 96 who were using various kinds of equipment were almost equally divided into two groups, 50 having had no difficulty in using it and 46 having experienced difficulties of various kinds. Typical problems they described included the following:

Wheelchairs:

1. Chairs are heavy to push and to lift into cars or put away in the house.

2. Folding chairs are difficult to fold. Some mothers were quite sure that their chairs were intended to fold but could not see how this had to be done. No one had instructed them as to how to handle the chairs.

3. When folded, the chairs are so large that even if the mother could manage to hold her child and to fold the chair at the same time, bus conductors will not allow them to be taken on ordinary service buses.

4. They are difficult to fit into cars or car boots. Some parents run a larger car than they would normally wish to run (e.g. a Ford Consul) to accommodate the chair. Others run vans, which will take the chair without folding.

   Some mothers suggested that a second, light chair, possibly made of canvas and easy to fold, would be invaluable and would enable them to make short bus journeys with their children, for example, to visit relatives, which at the moment were ruled out.[1]

5. Self-propelling chairs with very small wheels at the front are difficult to negotiate over kerbs and rough ground. Parents anxious to provide their children with a wide variety of outings, including country walks across the fields, often find this kind of activity very much hampered by the design of the chair.

6. It is difficult to carry shopping and push the chair at the same time.

7. Children are very exposed to the weather—very few chairs indeed are furnished with either hood or apron. Given the English climate, this is a limitation on use in all seasons.

8. Chairs with two handles are harder to push than those with a bar like an ordinary pram. The problem of folding the chair easily has to be reconciled with the need to make it as easy as possible to use.

9. Perhaps the greatest problem of all for mothers of children under five is the difficulty of providing a chair for the child who cannot use any of the pushchairs available commercially. These are not designed for large children who are still unable to sit up without support and who flop and slide in chairs which are adequate for normal children. Seven mothers mentioned this specifically when they were asked if there was anything they needed but could not get. Mothers have been told, they say, by the hospital almoner (who is one of the

---

[1] The 'Baby-Buggy', made by Andrews McLaren and on sale at a discount through the Spastics Society, is a lightweight push-chair which has been modified to meet the needs of young handicapped children. This firm is now working on a model for children older than 5.

various channels through which wheelchairs are obtained) that children are not eligible for chairs until they are at least 5 years old and that chairs are not made to fit children under 5. One said she was asked to pay the £35 that the chair cost herself, by the Local Executive Committee.

10. Making all possible allowance for faulty recollection, it nevertheless seems plain that considerable confusion exists both among parents and Health Service personnel as to the correct procedure for obtaining chairs. Perhaps no standardized procedure exists. When mothers were asked who had first advised them to obtain wheelchairs, replies included:

> The consultant in charge
> Orthopaedic consultant
> Local authority health visitor
> Spastics Society visitors
> Hospital sister
> Hospital almoner (medical social worker)
> Physiotherapist
> Special school personnel
> Maternity and child welfare clinic
> Other mothers

About a quarter of all mothers with wheelchairs pointed out that they had *asked* for them and that they felt that this was wrong—that it should not be left to them to judge the time to order essential equipment. Others said that they were not aware of the kinds of equipment available nor would they have known how to go about obtaining it. As one mother put it when she was asked 'Is there any gadget you would like to see made that you can't make yourselves?'—'I can't tell you duck, because I've never seen anything you *can* have.' Another mother, when asked: 'Is there anything you've asked for but haven't got?' replied, 'I don't know the place to go for anything—I've never been told, you know.' Yet another, when asked whether she would welcome more visits from social workers or home visitors, replied, 'Well, I don't think it'd help a lot, really. I should like to know more about what equipment they've got for spastics, you know, because—I mean, they only have to send out leaflets or something to show what equipment they *have* got, what you could get. But I've really no idea at all.'

Amesbury chairs (for indoor use)

In general, these chairs were praised by the 35 mothers who had them. However, some mothers complained that they were large and cumbersome and one that her chair had very small castors that made it difficult to move about on carpets. Another found the head supports or wings were in the wrong place for her child. One Amesbury chair was also a commode chair but the commode was described as 'wobbly' and too small.

One mother suggested that the chairs would be improved by having deeper sides to their trays so that cups, toys, etc., could not be so easily knocked off. She also suggested that interchangeable trays, to fit on the basic tray, could have holes of various shapes and sizes into which could be fitted bowls, toys, cups and anything else a child could use or play with. This might help to meet the criticism that some children soon become tired or bored in their chairs or simply 'don't like' them.

Large-size prams or spinal carriages

These tend to be unpopular because they are so long and ungainly, so that they are awkward to manoeuvre and mothers feel somewhat conspicuous with them. One mother had refused to accept one for these reasons.

Walking aids

Some kind of frame walker had been lent to 20 children. They were subject to specific criticisms relating to individual children; for example, certain children found the wheeled walkers difficult to control—they tended to 'run away' with the child. Another child could only go sideways with his walker, which had no wheels. They were also subject to the general criticism of weight, of being too heavy to be really manoeuvrable for a handicapped child.

One mother, who made this general criticism of all equipment— wheelchairs, calipers and aids of all kinds—had had a 'Rollator' walking aid copied in light alloy tubing, because she found the standard model in tubular steel too heavy for her child. He was very mobile with the lighter model both in the house and in the garden and could negotiate the back-door steps with it.

Since the survey has been completed, we have been informed[1] that the difficulties described under item 9 above should not have occurred because outdoor chairs for children aged 2 years have been available 'for at least ten years, if not more'. This means that this was the case during the time that the East Midlands mothers had reported difficulty on this point. We can only assume that some National Health Service personnel were

[1] By the Spastics Society, who had been in communication with the Assistant Director of Supply, Blackpool, on this subject.

unaware of the facts at the time. We have also been informed by the same source that any handicapped child or adult who needs a wheelchair both in and out of doors is entitled to have two chairs and that parents should insist upon such provision being made. Similarly, waterproof covers for chairs can be supplied on prescription. The Spastics Society is to publish in the near future a handbook for parents concerning the supply of equipment which will contain information about whom to approach when such equipment is required.

The fact that some of the difficulties need never have arisen highlights the communication problem that exists, concerning the dissemination of information to the parents of handicapped children and to personnel in the social services. This problem of communication has several different aspects, some of which will be discussed elsewhere in this book. As we have already pointed out, it seems, from the evidence obtained from the East Midlands mothers, that some members of the social services are not sufficiently well-informed about equipment available and how to get it. The proposals of the Seebohm Committee,[1] if adopted, could go some way towards channelling information more effectively. The number of East Midlands mothers who had experienced real difficulty in obtaining equipment was not large—about 10% of the 96 who had actually obtained the equipment eventually. However, among the mothers who had asked for equipment but had not got it, there were also some who had failed, it seemed, through confusion about who to get it from, although the majority eventually obtained what they needed, after some delay. Of the 51 mothers who had wheelchairs, for example, most had not waited longer than 5 months but 11 had waited 6 months or longer. However, it is hard to understand why the mother of a 6-year-old should have had the experience described below, which she recounted when asked whether she had a wheelchair for her child.

The physiotherapist arranged the Amesbury chair for me and then the wheelchair—of course, that has to be through a doctor. She advised me to go to my own doctor but they looked through their catalogues and they hadn't got one small enough at that time and of course I had to ask Dr —— (the consultant). He arranged for me to see the almoner at the hospital. Of course, she rang through

[1] See the report of the *Committee on Local Authority and Allied Personal Social Services* (The Seebohm Report), Cmmd. 3703 H.M.S.O., London 1968.

to both the County and the Ministry of Pensions[1]—because this particular chair we've got, they make a smaller one than the other (firm) and there's only the Ministry of Pensions have them so she got it through that.

The next mother had a child of 3 and was interviewed in 1966.

I tried to get one (wheelchair) but they wouldn't let me have one, they said she wasn't old enough. (Interviewer: Who told you she wasn't old enough?) The almoner at the hospital. Dr —— (the consultant) thought we should have one for her . . . a pushchair's not big enough for her, she just slides straight out of the bottom. She'll have to be about 5 before she can have one.

It is apparent that it is not always easy to insist on one's rights in this respect. It is not even easy to act independently and buy equipment privately. The mother of a 3-year-old girl asked the consultant if her child would benefit from using an Amesbury chair. He suggested she ask the Spastics Society home visitor about getting one. The home visitor passed the request to the local authority health department, who informed the mother that the funds allocated for this kind of help had been exhausted. She said she was willing to pay for the chair herself if the department would tell her who to get in touch with. She was informed that this was not known. She heard of an exhibition being held in town, showing equipment for the disabled but arrived to find it had finished, having lasted only two days. She said, 'If only I knew *where* to get one—I'll buy it. We do try to help ourselves'.

Two other mothers in similar situations contacted members of parliament, one without success, the other (who wrote to the Prime Minister) with spectacular success but not all parents are willing to go to such lengths. They should not need to.

Mothers were asked whether their husbands and/or friends or relatives had been able to make any gadgets or equipment for their children themselves. Fifty-four (30%) replied that they had and described a wide variety of things. Forty-two (23%) had never found it necessary to do so and the remaining 47% replied that they had not done so, often commenting that their husbands were not good at that kind of thing or that they were not able to conceive of anything that would help.

---

[1] This may be an example of confusion on the mother's part about which department is responsible for wheelchairs. The Ministry of Health was responsible for their provision at the time of interview. (This is now the Ministry of Health and Social Security.)

The fathers (or other relatives) who were talented handymen and who could obtain materials and tools (or the help of skilled workmen at work) were able to alter and adapt pushchairs, beds and babychairs to suit their own children. The problem of pushchairs has already been discussed above. A similar problem arises with beds, when children grow out of their cots and are not safe in ordinary beds. Mothers described the difficulty experienced in trying to buy beds with adequate sides at reasonable cost. Two local authorities had helped two mothers by lending large metal hospital cots, to cope with very active, mentally handicapped children. The father of another very active, mentally handicapped little girl of three, who was very big for her age and who fell constantly, had designed and made a beautifully padded play-pen and a bed with padded sides—one side formed by the wall of the room. One mother found that the firm 'Myers' will supply a bed with adequate side rails, if specially requested, but these beds are not cheap.

The problem of car seats similar to those made for babies but large enough for older children was frequently mentioned. Some fathers had managed to alter bought seats, others had improvised and produced their own models; but when mothers were asked if there were any gadgets they would like that they could not make themselves, car seats were mentioned several times.

In addition to large items like wheelchairs, there are many gadgets and modifications to ordinary household equipment which can help the handicapped child and his mother to overcome difficulties with the everyday activities of eating, toiletting and bathing. These aids to daily living are not supplied as of right, through the National Health Service but, as with modifications to homes, welfare departments of the local authority have powers to assist in their provision. These departments should also be able to advise parents about ways to make such gadgets themselves.

Several fathers in the East Midlands sample had modified the handles of spoons and forks. One mother said that the materials to do this had been supplied by the physiotherapist. Others mentioned it as something they wanted to do but could not think how to do it or where to get the appropriate materials.

Bathing a large, helpless child is very difficult. Many mothers solve the problem by enlisting the help of other members of the family, often to the extent of getting one of the other children to bath with the handicapped child and support him. Four mothers said that something to help support their children in the bath would be a great help[1] and one wanted a bath lift or hoist to get him in and out of the bath.

A solution to the problem of supporting the child in the water had been devised by one mother; she had got a carpenter to fix a rail to a rafter in the bathroom ceiling, over the bath, along which ran a wheel. The baby bouncer was fixed to the wheel and the child could be supported in the bouncer and swished backwards and forwards in the bath.

Some of the most trying difficulties, however, are those which cannot be alleviated by the proper supply of wheelchairs or other aids to daily living. The mother of a child who is difficult to get to sleep has only her own resourcefulness to help her. This problem was by no means common to the majority of the sample—more than half the mothers had never had any difficulty. Fifty-two (29%) were still having difficulty at the time of interview and the 24 mothers (13%) who had coped with this problem in the past had no difficulty in recalling how hard it had been to bear. The remedy was often to keep the child up until the whole family went to bed or to nurse or soothe the child to sleep in some way. This was also necessary for some of the normal 4-year-olds and the subject of bedtime is discussed in detail in Chapter 4 where the experience of the two samples is compared. One point which it is important to remember is that the handicapped children seemed less likely to be able to 'comfort' themselves to sleep than are normal children. The normal 4-year-olds, for example, made greater use of 'transitional objects' such as cloths or pieces of old blanket and they sucked thumbs, bottles and dummies more often than did the handicapped children. A mother whose child had needed comfort when she was small describes how she used to soothe this very handicapped little girl, 5 years old:

She used to scream and scream, day and night. We never knew what it was to have an hour's sleep with her. When she was tiny

[1] There is now a more suitable bath seat—the 'Safa-seat'—available commercially and through the Spastics Society. This seat and several more practical solutions to bath-time problems are illustrated in *Handling the Young Cerebral Palsied Child at Home*, by Nancie R. Finnie, M.C.S.P., Heinemann Medical Books, London, 1968.

and she used to yell so much, we'd brush her hair and she would be quiet while ever you kept doing it. I used to say we ought to have an automatic hair brush in bed! We used to take a hair brush to bed, always.

The mother who speaks next[1] had found life impossible because her son was such a poor sleeper as a baby and as a young child.

He's a lot better than he was. We were frantic for 8 years. That's one of the reasons why we wanted residential care for him, because we'd never had a night's sleep for 8 years. He used to go to bed and he used to cry and shout—oh, for 2 or 3 hours. At the time it got to such a pitch that I just couldn't cope any longer and we found it was affecting the whole family, you know—it just wasn't being a unit any more. I was tired, my husband was tired, we were irritable and snapping at (the unhandicapped child). We find now he is away that we look forward to the holidays and we'll enjoy them and he does seem to be a lot better now . . . As I say, most nights he does wake up . . . we've reached the stage now where we just change beds. I laugh about it but I was really frantic, you know. It got to such a pitch that I resented him. It was a horrible thing—I loved him and yet I resented him for the ill-feeling and unhappiness he was causing the rest of us, you know.

Twenty-one children were having some kind of sedation at bedtime but it was not always clear from the mothers' accounts whether this was part of their anti-convulsant therapy or simply to control their sleeping difficulties.

Feeding difficulties can also worry mothers greatly. These occur quite frequently with normal children. However, with normal children the problem is not that they cannot eat but that they *will* not eat or are highly selective about what they will eat. In this last respect, the cerebral palsied and the normal 4-year-old children were very similar—70% of the handicapped children were considered to be good eaters, as were 61% of the 4-year-olds; 17% of the handicapped were 'finicky' about what they would eat and so were 14% of the 4-year-olds. For the cerebral palsied children, the real problem is more likely to be that of finding a way to teach them to chew and swallow so that they can move on from the soft foods of their baby days to a

[1] This mother was not included in the 180 whose replies were finally analysed. As her child was no longer living at home, he was not eligible for inclusion. However, she wanted to be interviewed and had some interesting comments to make on several topics.

more normal diet. Twenty-six of the East Midlands children, aged from 1 year to 8 years, could still take only minced or mashed foods, 16 aged from 1 year to 7 years could take only liquids or puréed baby foods, and 4 aged from 2 years to 5 years were still completely bottle-fed. Some mothers who worried that their children's diet might be deficient in protein because their children were unable to chew meat, were buying them extra milk or milk foods such as Horlicks or Complan and others bought Heinz baby foods. A very small number had been provided with special 'Mouli' graters or liquidisers in order to purée foods themselves. The extra cost of special foods was sometimes mentioned as a problem, but more important, in most cases, is the extra time it takes to feed a child who cannot chew and swallow normally. There are various techniques that can be employed that will help to overcome these difficulties, but there was no evidence from the East Midlands mothers that they had received practical instruction on how to employ such techniques. The mothers quoted below were at different stages in the process of tackling the problem—one was still trying, one had virtually given up and the third had a child who was receiving therapy in which the mother had not been asked to participate.

Boy: 1 yr.

I tried him with one of these drip cups—you know, with a hole at the side—but he can't drink, he can't do it and if he gets too much he chokes, you see . . . the other day I had a terrible fright with him. I gave him cornflakes, I squeezed the cornflakes up and put hot milk on—I thought 'They'll not choke him' and he got some at the back of his throat. We had a terrible job with him. I thought 'No more—it's the last time I'm going to give him them!' I tried him on Heinz junior foods—'cos he has strained (foods) all the time, you see—but he can't take it, he was sick. I've tried and tried him with everything—I've done everything with him but he just can't do it. He can't take it, no matter what I do.

Boy: 6 yrs.

He won't eat potatoes—we've tried all ways. He has a good breakfast, he likes porridge; but he won't eat his dinner. At one time he would eat custard but not now. *We just give him what he likes— ice cream and chocolate drops and things.* When he goes away from home he won't eat at all.

Girl: 7 yrs.

Well, apparently she wasn't chewing properly when she went to school (where she is a five-day boarder). They've been giving her chewing therapy and she now chews better. I don't know how they do this—mouth exercises, I think, to encourage them to chew properly.

Twenty-one mothers had found that feeding was their greatest problem. Thirty-six mothers usually gave the handicapped child his meals separately from the rest of the family for various reasons but the majority of children shared family mealtimes in spite of difficulties.

Sixty-seven children (38%) were doubly incontinent and 44 of them were over 5 years old. We were therefore surprised when only 8 mothers gave this as their greatest problem. Nappy-washing is apparently more easily accepted than other aspects of caring for handicapped children. Some mothers had found difficulty in obtaining large enough nappies and waterproof pants. When found, these had proved to be expensive. Attempts to toilet-train some of these children had met with little success. It is difficult to tell when a child's level of understanding is sufficient for him to know what is expected of him when he is regularly sat on his potty or the toilet. If children respond to attempts at training by screaming and struggling, it is hard to know whether they are frightened, suffering pain or discomfort or whether they simply do not understand what is happening. They may be frightened by the toilet but unable to explain their fear. Spastic children may stiffen uncontrollably when they are sat down in unfamiliar surroundings or on uncomfortable, insecure seats or potties. It is extremely unrewarding for mothers to persist with toilet training in these circumstances. In some ways, it is easier to give up and resign oneself to washing nappies.

Boy: 8 yrs.

He's in nappies. That's my big problem with him. We've only got an upstairs toilet—and he's very heavy. I used to have a commode and he just used to stiffen out, he just used to sit and scream and he wouldn't use it. I'm hoping that when they get him into a school that they can clear that up for me because he won't do it for me.

Boy: 5 yrs.

I don't think I could make him sit on the toilet even if I had a chair, we have thought about it once or twice. What we could do with is a special kind of potty but I can't get one that is really comfortable. If you take him up to the toilet you may be sat struggling with him so long. I've brought that (large mirror) down from the bathroom, I've found that he'll use his potty when he's sat in front of that. We used to put one on the table when he was just learning to feed himself and he used to sit longer—when he's done his hair he likes to look through the mirror at himself.

This mother's use of the mirror is interesting and may be a useful suggestion that others might try. Children are always interested in how they look when they are doing things—the children who come to the playroom at Nottingham's Child Development Research Unit are sometimes more fascinated at first with watching themselves in the large mirror that forms the one-way vision screen than by all the toys in the room, particularly if there are no other children in the room. However, the main difficulty with toilet training, as with feeding, is the time it takes. The only really practical book on caring for cerebral palsied children[1] that has yet been published in England suggests that 'The best way of tackling the problem of toilet training is to "pot" your child every hour when he is at home even though he may no longer be a baby.' This may not be very realistic advice to a busy mother who has everything to do for the rest of her family as well as caring for her handicapped child. However, most of the advice contained in this book is very practical indeed. Something is suggested for every problem we have noted above, including ways to handle children during bathing, dressing and feeding, that will help to counteract the unhelpful movement patterns that can hinder these activities.

How to enable a handicapped child to play as he needs to is another area where many mothers would welcome helpful suggestions. Nancie Finnie's book again is a mine of information, but, as with everything else, it is time above all that a mother needs in order to attend to her child's play activities.

When we asked mothers what kind of toys their children most liked to play with and what was their favourite occupation, their replies seemed to indicate that mental handicap is an important factor. If this is severe, it limits the child's ability to play, even when physical handicaps are slight. Twenty children who had mental handicaps or whose mental status had to be classified as uncertain, were said by their mothers not to enjoy

[1] Finnie, Nancie, op. cit.

any activity at all. These children varied in age from 2 to 7 years. Others, again of all ages, were interested only in the sounds of rattles, newspaper being rattled or torn, or squeaky toys. Children of normal or apparently normal intelligence, on the other hand, seemed able to exercise great ingenuity in amusing themselves, particularly if they had good hand control. Functional mobility[1] is important, too. For 23 children (13% of the sample) this appeared to be unaffected by their handicaps. Twenty others (11%) were restricted a little but were able to go out to play in the street or the park. Ten more could get to neighbouring houses to play with friends or take messages.

A tricycle with blocks on the pedals and a supporting back rest is a great help to some children who can walk only slowly. One 6-year-old boy in the pilot sample, who could not walk at all unaided, had, within a month of acquiring such a tricycle, extended his horizons from the four walls of a farmhouse kitchen to the neighbours' houses at the other end of the lane, thus many times multiplying his social as well as his geographical experiences.

Another boy, 8 years old and determined to ride a two-wheeled bicycle, had taught himself to do this in spite of the fact that he found it very difficult to balance. He was sufficiently lightly handicapped to be able to compete in games with normal children, but his handicaps did make it hard for him to succeed. His mother described his problem vividly:

He'll sail through sports day until it's over and then he's heart-broken because he couldn't win anything. He loves sport, that's the unfortunate part. He reckoned he wouldn't play football and cricket and that sort of thing, but I've coached him—if you show them the best way to cope with it, with his handicap, it's surprising what he can do. We always set out to help him in those ways, because we tell him there isn't such a word as can't. There's always a way. But they told him at the hospital he'd never ride a two-wheeled bike, his balance is so bad. And we had quite a 'to-do' last summer when our other little boy got on a friend's bike and rode it straight away. He was heartbroken. He came in and cried in the chair. I said to him 'Now, look, you've told me you want a bike. It's no good me buying one if you can't ride it, so get off out there, get on it and ride it. You can do it.' An hour later he came in—he was cuts and bruises, poor bairn, all over,

[1] Defined in Chapter 1.

but he'd mastered it. It's agony to watch him, bless him, how he does it I don't know, but the point is he's mastered it. He can't ride one well, I'm not going to say he can, but the point is he can ride a bike. That sort of gave him confidence and we have got him a bike now.

Really difficult problems arise for those who are mentally and physically handicapped and chair-bound as well. One such boy, aged 8½ years liked tearing paper, playing with plastic buses, turning the pages of books (several mothers mentioned mail-order catalogues as being favourites with their children), playing with his teddy-bear and listening to music. A girl aged 6 mostly played with building bricks and dolls, while sitting in her chair. At the time of interview, she was not attending a day centre or nursery centre and although she was one of a very large family, the other children usually went out to play. Her mother said she would not move around or do anything when she was put on the floor. Children such as these, seem to need to be taught how to play, and their mothers need to be taught how to help them do this. Again, Nancie Finnie's book[1] is full of ideas, but 'toy-centres', where mothers could take the children to try out various kinds of toys and ways of playing with them before committing themselves to expensive purchases, would be of great value. One such centre already in existence is the Enfield 'Noah's Ark' Toy Library.[2] This very successful enterprise specializes in lending toys which have been proved to be of value in helping handicapped children of all kinds, not only to enjoy themselves but also to extend their opportunities for learning.

We asked mothers what they thought was the child's greatest handicap, from his point of view. The majority (67%) emphasized different aspects and consequences of physical disabilities. Thirty-nine (22%) thought lack of speech or difficulty in communicating hampered children more than anything else. Only 16 (9%) put mental handicap first. Five mothers felt that their children's disabilities were so minimal that they were not really handicapped in any way.

We then asked mothers what it was about the child that they

[1] Op. cit.
[2] Brochure and literature available from: Enfield 'Noah's Ark' Toy Library, 21 Gentleman's Row, Enfield, Middlesex, on receipt of 6d. stamped, addressed foolscap envelope.

found most difficult to cope with. We have mentioned three of these problems earlier in the chapter—carrying and lifting, 36 mothers (20%); incontinence, 8 mothers (4%); feeding difficulties, 21 mothers (12%). Seventeen mothers (9%) found difficulty in communicating with their children their greatest problem and 5 (3%) mentioned difficulties related to the child's mental handicap. Thirty mothers could think of nothing that was particularly hard to deal with. Most of their children (24) were not severely handicapped. It was interesting to find that over a third of the replies to this question were so highly individual, that they could not be conveniently included in general categories. Difficulties mentioned ranged from trying aspects of the child's temperament—'moodiness', 'mardiness', 'temper tantrums,' 'being miserable', 'disobedience'—to practical difficulties that stemmed from physical disabilities. Several mothers stressed the child's total helplessness and dependence. Others could think of only relatively minor aspects of caring for their children—'washing her hair', 'messiness at table'—or their children's general slowness in everyday activities. Such things may seem trivial to an onlooker, but they can be very trying to deal with day after day over a long period of time. There were practical difficulties, such as the amount of laundry, the expense of buying shoes as frequently as every 3 or 4 weeks and the search for *suitable* shoes—'it costs you a fortune in clothes alone.' The mother of a very severely handicapped boy, who had other children, said: 'It's not the trouble, but *time*', and a few mothers found it very hard to bear when their children suffered social consequences of their handicap. Other children would not play with them, or they could not meet other children on equal terms. The mother of such a child said that the worst thing, to her, was 'him getting upset about being handicapped. There's so little you can do to comfort him'.

In addition to attending to the daily needs of their children, it usually falls to the mother's lot to take the children to hospital out-patient clinics for their medical supervision. Some children also have to be taken every week for physiotherapy or speech therapy. Only 26 mothers (14% of the sample) said that their children were not having any medical supervision.

Eight children (4%) were seen by doctors at school. Some of their parents had been told that they would be informed when medical examinations were to take place so that they might attend but in practice this did not seem to happen, except in one instance. This child attended a special day school in a city area and was examined at school once a term. The mother was present at these examinations and found them satisfactory. The mother of another child attending the same school, thought he was examined every month, but she was not sure of this and had never been asked to examinations.

Fifty-nine (40%) of the mothers who attended consultants' clinics at hospital, reported no difficulties in keeping appointments. The most frequently reported difficulty was the length of time spent waiting to see the doctor (41 mothers). A long wait is particularly trying for handicapped children, and some mothers felt that a better organized appointments system would be beneficial for everyone, including the doctors, who have to examine children who have become tired and irritable after a long wait. Canteen or coffee bar facilities are very much appreciated where they exist and regretted when they have been closed. Hot drink vending machines do not adequately replace such services.

Facilities for changing large-size incontinent children would also help. At one hospital, children have to be carried up about 50 stone stairs to the Children's Department, a difficulty with large, helpless children. Waiting rooms and seating are still inadequate in some hospitals—some mothers commented that they realized that there is not unlimited money available for such amenities but they would certainly appreciate having their task made a little less difficult. Most of them are very conscientious about keeping their appointments, even when they feel that there is little reward in their short interview with the doctor after a long and uncomfortable wait.

Twenty mothers complained of the ambulance services. Again, they were very ready to make allowances for the obvious difficulties of running such a service but the time of these mothers is so precious, especially when they have other children, that they are bound to resent having to wait for transport, often till long past children's normal meal times. The difficulty here stems mainly from the fact that ambulances have to be shared by several patients in order to run the service at all. This means considerable time is spent in touring round to pick everyone up. Mothers have to be ready and waiting to go whenever the ambulance arrives. This is inconvenient enough when they are waiting at home for the journey to hospital. Often the most trying time comes after they have seen the doctor and are waiting to go home again.

Ten mothers experienced difficulty travelling by public transport. Eight of them lived in rural areas and their difficulties included the problem of getting child and pushchair on and off buses. Time was a factor, too—even in a city it can take 1 to $1\frac{1}{2}$ hours to reach the hospital when it is necessary to take more than one bus.

Eight mothers had problems getting someone to look after their other children while they attended hospital. Five of them had been forced to break some appointments when relatives who usually came to look after the children could not do so. Two of the fathers of these 8 children took time off from work to solve this problem.

Almost half the children (81, or 45%) attended at other times for physiotherapy and/or speech therapy.

Nine children (5%) were having speech therapy, 4 of them at school.

Seventy-six children were having some physiotherapy. Thirteen of these were receiving their treatment at school or day centre and a further 3 were visited at home by the therapist. For the mothers of these 16 children there were obviously no problems of travelling or waiting.

Of the 60 children attending hospitals or clinics for physiotherapy, none had experienced the problem of a lengthy wait before going in to the therapist, a tribute to the organization of appointments and in marked contrast to mothers' experience in relation to paediatrician and other specialist clinics. The explanation is probably that it is much easier for a physiotherapist to restrict her case-load to the number it is physically possible for her to handle, than it is for a doctor to estimate how long he will need to spend with any one referral.

The ambulance service for taking children to treatment was criticized by 6 mothers only, who had experienced long waits for transport. Six more mothers had experienced difficulty travelling to appointments, but the majority (56) reported no particular difficulties in keeping their appointments.

Since the strain of meeting the needs of their handicapped children without neglecting the rest of the family falls mainly on the mothers, it would not be surprising to find that their physical and mental well-being was impaired because of this. We asked the East Midlands mothers whether they considered themselves to be in good health and also whether they suffered from feelings of depression. (There are no comparable data for the normal sample.) Their replies are set out in Table 3.III. Almost half the sample considered themselves to be in good health, and these were equally divided into those who often felt depressed, and those who did not. Not surprisingly, mothers whose health is not good are significantly[1] more likely to say that they also feel depressed. We asked the mothers who said that they were 'nervy', 'run-down' or 'depressed' whether they had been to their family doctors about this. Forty-three of them said that there was no point in doing so because they did not expect general practitioners to be very understanding about this kind of condition. They felt they were expected to deal with their depression without help. Some mothers felt that the cause

TABLE 3.III

| | Mothers' state of health | | | | |
	Good	Moderate	Run-down	Poor	Total
Depression emphasized	43 (24%)	31 (17%)	13 (7%)	22 (12%)	109 (61%)
No particular emphasis on depression	41 (23%)	18 (10%)	8 (5%)	4 (2%)	71 (39%)
Total	84 (47%)	49 (27%)	21 (12%)	26 (14%)	180 (100%)

of their depression was that they were with their handicapped children so much without any relief (see Table 6.I for school and day-care provision). Day centres for all children, including pre-school children, would help to relieve this situation. The mothers who went out to work found that this improved their morale, because they were able, for a short time, to live without being constantly reminded of their troubles, and this more than offset the extra effort and fatigue of being in paid employment.

Relief for hard-pressed mothers is provided through local authority mental welfare departments, with the co-operation of

[1] When the two small groups who said their health was 'poor' or that they felt very 'run down' were combined, this trend was consistent.
$$\chi^2 = 6\cdot0 \quad \eta = 2 \quad \text{Significant at } \cdot05 \text{ level.}$$

hospitals for the mentally sub-normal. The Family Help Units set up by the Spastics Society also offer temporary residential care for any cerebral palsied child, although difficulties arise here over the cost of providing such care. Arrangements can sometimes be made with local authorities for them to meet such costs, but where authorities believe their own provision to be adequate, they are of course, reluctant to pay for the services of a voluntary society.

Temporary care of some kind had been accepted at least once by 73 mothers (41%). A further 25 (14%) expressed willingness to accept this if it were offered. Thirty-one mothers (17%), mainly of the lightly handicapped, felt no need for relief of this kind, and another 51 (28%) would not consider it for other reasons.

Among those who had accepted such help were some who said they would not do so a second time, and others with many reservations about it. A criticism of the care provided by hospitals for the subnormal, was that such care was usually arranged for periods of 3 or 4 weeks at a time. Mothers felt that this seemed a long time both to themselves and to the children. Some mothers also said that they were given such short notice of the actual dates during which the handicapped child would be cared for, that they were unable to make holiday arrangements for the rest of the family, thus partly defeating the purpose of short-term care. The standards of care in these hospitals were occasionally criticized by a minority of mothers who described how their children had lost weight during their stay and returned home with bruises or with sores on their faces and bedsores on their backs and buttocks. Others described how their children had pined, particularly if parents had been advised not to visit. This last point also applied to the Family Help Unit in Nottingham[1] and is well expressed in the following quotation:

> *They* reckoned he settled very well. You couldn't visit him that month he was away because of upsetting me and upsetting him and they reckon he was very happy and that, but he definitely lost weight. Well, I think myself was pining. I mean, for a *normal* child to be suddenly took from his mother is a crime, isn't it?

[1] Since this survey was completed, we have been informed by the Family Help Unit that parents are now advised that children may be visited freely, at all times, during their stay there. Parents who are away on holiday, obviously cannot visit, nor can those who have had to have their children cared for because they are ill themselves.

Nothing to say about the Mount, mind you, and the person in charge is marvellous. And the whole place itself was a lovely place, beautiful from top to bottom, but I don't think I'd let him go there again. Every 3 months he can go, but we won't let him go. It's only now, this last week, he's got back to normal. When we fetched him out he'd forgotten everything we'd learnt him and he was just . . . frightened, you know.

This little boy was 2 years old, but similar comments were made about older children. On the other hand, other mothers had nothing but praise for the Family Help Unit or the hospitals and described how much their children had improved during their stay.

There are certain aspects of this problem which create difficulty. Although it is now generally acknowledged that young children in hospital need to maintain regular contact with their mothers, this may not be so obvious with children who are in theory old enough, in years, to tolerate separations reasonably well, but who are developmentally still very young. This could be particularly true of mentally retarded children who may not be able to understand why they are separated from their families, nor that this separation is only temporary. Such children may actually need to be visited more frequently than normal children, not less.

It is possible, too, that a short stay at the Family Help Unit may seem to some parents to be in a different category from a stay in hospital. These parents would probably visit a sick child in hospital as a matter of course, even if the child cried when they had to go away again. Both hospital personnel and parents are beginning to understand that it may be better for the young child, in the long term, to be upset by visiting than to be completely out of touch with his mother while he is away from home. A stay in the Family Help Unit may seem to be a different situation. The Unit's atmosphere is as home-like as possible, the child is not sick and is not undergoing treatment. Nevertheless, he *is* separated from his mother, his family and his home. From the young child's point of view, the two experiences may not be very different.

On the other hand, it is often essential that the mothers of handicapped children and possibly the rest of the family should be given some respite from caring for them. There is a genuine conflict of interest here.

In all families, a problem arises when an emergency necessitates the mother's temporary absence from home. We asked the East Midlands mothers who would care for the children if they were suddenly called away, or had to go into hospital without warning. Table 3.IV gives their replies.

TABLE 3.IV

Emergency care

Type of care	For CP child (N=180)	For the other children in the family (N=142)
Father would take time off work	23 (13%)	31 (22%)
Father and/or other relatives	67 (37%)	92 (65%)
Father and/or friends and neighbours	10 (6%)	18 (9%)
Institutional care (including the Family Help Unit)*	78 (43%)	5 (4%)
Don't know	2 (1%)	1
		142
Families with no sibs or adult sibs only		38
	180 (100%)	180 (100%)

* Fifty-four mothers mentioned the Family Help Unit by name; 15 mentioned local authority provision, 6 did not know how such care would be arranged; the almoner, the paediatrician and the school where the child was a 5-day boarder were mentioned once each as the agencies through which some care of some kind would be obtained.

For the normal siblings, the crisis could be met almost completely by the family. Relatives and friends would help by taking one of the children or by minding young school-age children until their fathers came home from work. Of the 5 mothers who could not rely on family help for the normal children, 1 had a husband who was mentally ill and relatives who would not help, 1 was Indian and without relatives in England, 1 had 8 children and very little contact with relatives, 1 had marital problems and the last could rely on her daily help to have the child.

The proportion of families who could cope with the handicapped child is only a little more than half that of the normal children. Fifty-six per cent of the spastic children could be cared for within the family or with the help of friends and neighbours and 43% would probably need to ask the help of the Family Help Unit or some other institution, whereas 96% of the normal siblings could be cared for within the family. This is the consequence both of the lack of confidence in their own capabilities sometimes felt by relatives[1] and of the reluctance of parents to ask others to accept the extra responsibilities involved in caring for children who are difficult to feed, bath, dress and care for generally.

We have so far discussed aspects of caring for handicapped children that cost time and effort. Sometimes there are extra financial burdens as well. Although only 13 mothers (7%) mentioned financial help when asked if there was any kind of help they would have liked that they had not had, many more mentioned in passing that extra expense had been incurred for the handicapped child. Shoes were a problem for those who dragged their feet. The knees of trousers wear out very quickly when children crawl. Dribbling spoils the front of sweaters and dresses. Large size nappies and waterproof pants are expensive. So are the special foods that mothers feel they must provide for children with difficulty in chewing and swallowing. Travelling expenses can be quite heavy when children in hospital have to be visited. Sometimes several push-chairs have to be bought for the handicapped child when one would have been adequate for a normal child.

When such expenses as these are considered, a case can be made for the payment of a special children's allowance to be made to mothers of handicapped children, particularly to those who have no day-care for their young children and to those who continue to care for their older children instead of accepting permanent residential care for them. These parents make their contribution to society through rates and taxes but they get a poor return when their children do not go to school or to a day centre. These same children cannot use the parks, the libraries and the swimming baths. An allowance would be a small token of society's recognition that mothers are doing a very difficult job that would cost a great deal if it had to be taken over by the state. Precise statements of the cost of keeping children in subnormality hospitals, which are the institutions most likely to care for the kind of child we are discussing, are not easy to come

[1] See Chapter 5, page 124.

by but the Ministry of Health in its Annual Report for 1966/67[1] gives the average cost of maintaining these hospitals as £11 11s 7d per inpatient-week, this figure including adult and child patients. Although this figure is considerably lower than that for other kinds of hospital care (it is soon to be made more nearly comparable to the figure for psychiatric hospital care), it affords some measure of the goods and services received by a mother whose handicapped child is cared for in hospital and, conversely, of those supplied by a mother who continues to care for her equally handicapped child at home.

[1] Cmmd. 3702 H.M.S.O.

CHAPTER 4

THE EFFECTS OF HANDICAP ON
PATTERNS OF FAMILY LIFE

*It is no exaggeration to say that in the background of
every individual handicapped child there is always a
handicapped family.*

MARY SHERIDAN[1]

One of our main concerns in this study of handicapped children,
has been to attempt to discover the extent to which the lives of
their families differ from the lives of families which include only
normal children. References to the adverse effects of handicap
on the family are only too easy to find in the literature, and the
conviction that serious disruption of internal family relationships, and of relationships with the outside world are inevitable
concomitants of handicap seems to have been received into the
'conventional wisdom' almost without question. A recent mani-
festation of this phenomenon appeared in an article in one of
the more reputable of our Sunday newspapers,[2] which described
a new centre for the ˜erebral palsied and their families. The
relevant paragraph is quoted almost in its entirety, because it is
virtually an 'omnibus edition' of the ills which may befall the
'handicapped' family:

'Without adequate help, the birth of a handicapped child can
be the final straw that breaks a marriage apart. Often the other
children in a family with a spastic child are in danger emotionally
because the handicapped member of the family is given all the
love and attention. Less frequently, just the opposite happens:
the handicapped child is regarded as a "failure" and any other
children in the family will be pushed too hard and expected to
excel as compensation. Invariably the family of a handicapped

---

[1] Sheridan, Mary, *The Handicapped Child and his Home*. National Children's
Home, London, 1965.
[2] *The Sunday Times*. London, March 31, 1968.

child goes through feelings of guilt, resentment, confusion, despair and, above all, isolation.'

Add to this list a recent research finding that if such families do not break down there is a strong possibility that they will be 'too cohesive'[1] and include the danger that the handicapped children will be 'over-dependent' because their mothers are 'over-protective'[2] and the catalogue of ills is formidable indeed.

For several reasons, it is not easy to discuss concepts such as guilt and overprotectiveness and the pathological family reactions we have referred to. They appear in the literature often without careful definition, presumably because it is assumed that everyone will know what they mean and will use them in the same way. When, for example, parents are referred to as feeling guilty about their handicapped child, it is often unclear whether the person writing means that they feel guilty because they have produced a handicapped child; because they cannot feel the same way about him as they would if he were not handicapped; because they are not doing enough for him; because they are doing *too* much for him; because they want to send him away from home; because they want to keep him at home, or because they are neglecting their other children—or all of these at once. This somewhat elusive guilt is then related by some writers to the equally elusive concept of overprotectiveness and its correlative overdependence. To quote Dr Sheridan again,[3] 'It is a common reaction on the part of many affectionate and well-meaning parents to overprotect their child. It is sometimes said that this attitude stems from two different roots. The first originates in deep compassion so that parents feel they must try to make up to him, by over-indulgence and protection from unhappiness or discomfort, for all the ordinary experiences he has been denied. The second is rooted in their own feelings of guilt or warped self-pity, which they attempt to assuage by over-solicitousness for his welfare.' The consensus of opinion is that these parental attitudes will adversely affect the psychological development of the handicapped child and possibly that of his brothers and sisters as well.

Although evidence is available that suggests that the problem

[1] Schaffer, H. R. 'The Too-cohesive Family—a Form of Group Pathology'. *The International Journal of Social Psychiatry*, Vol. X, No. 4, 1964.
[2] Schonell, F. Eleanor. *Educating Spastic Children*. Edinburgh, 1957.
[3] Op. cit.

of undesirable parental attitudes has been exaggerated, this is not often acknowledged in the literature on cerebral palsy. A notable exception is Helle Neilson's careful review of research findings on all aspects of cerebral palsy.[1] Dr Howard R. Kelman[2] also reviews the origins of the consensus on parental attitude and concludes that unjustifiable generalizations have been made from evidence gathered in clinical situations from unrepresentative samples. Boles,[3] reporting on his controlled study of 60 mothers of cerebral palsied children, said 'While one might be inclined to think only of the parents of a child with a problem as anxious, guilty, unrealistic and rejecting, the findings of this study point otherwise and clearly suggest that attitudes of this type may exist generally, in marked degree, in our culture.' The culture referred to is that of the U.S.A. Evidence that our own culture may engender similar attitudes in parents of normal children came to light during the survey of normal 4-year-olds in Nottingham.[4] More than half of the mothers interviewed were critical of themselves in their maternal role and they frequently expressed feelings of guilt because of failure to be the sort of mother they considered to be ideal.

Some support for Dr Kelman's view (see above) is given by Dr A. I. Roith,[5] a consultant psychiatrist. Speaking of parents of mentally subnormal children, he says that the literature gives 'a completely biased and prejudiced impression of these parents'. He 'sat back and waited for the horde of guilty and aggressive parents to descend upon him' and after eight years was still waiting. Dr Sheridan[6] suggests that it might be 'more generous if, in the future, we omitted the term 'guilt complex' not only from our discussions but from our thoughts. If parents feel guilty, it may be that we ourselves have been the cause, because we have implied that they have every reason to feel guilty.'

In addition to these considerations, there is the difficulty that

[1] Neilson, Helle H. *A Psychological Study of Cerebral Palsied Children.* Munksgaard, Copenhagen, 1966.

[2] Kelman, Howard R. 'The Brain-damaged Child and his Family', in Birch, Herbert G. (Ed.). *Brain Damage in Children—the Biological and Social Aspects.* Williams & Wilkins, Baltimore, 1964.

[3] Boles, G. 'Personality Factors in Mothers of Cerebral Palsied Children'. *Genet. Psychol. Monogr.*, 1959, **59**, 159–218.

[4] Newson, J. & E., 1964. Op. cit.

[5] Roith, A. I. 'The Myth of Parental Attitudes'. *The Journal of Mental Subnormality*, 1963, **9**, 51–54.

[6] Op. cit.

systematic information about the behaviour of 'normal' or 'ordinary' families is hard to come by. It is difficult even to decide what is meant by the term 'ordinary' family[1] but unless such information can be made available, it is not possible to tell how much the so-called handicapped families deviate from the norm. We need to know more of the families who never come under the searchlight of the clinician or the case-worker.

Not only are the concepts of parental attitudes and family states elusive, it is also difficult to decide how to judge their applicability to any one family. There is no doubt that in using these concepts professional people are passing judgement on parents and the judgement is not a favourable one. Beatrice Wright[2] has pointed out that the concept of over-protection is 'part and parcel of the cultural value placed on dependence and independence' and she presents a very interesting discussion of the possibility of using apparently objective criteria for judging 'over-protection' when one is already proclaiming one's bias by the very use of such a term, which has in-built notions of undesirability. The point at which reasonable care of children becomes over-protection is difficult enough to establish with any degree of justice or accuracy, even when the child is normal. Two dimensions of the problem have to be considered—on the one hand, there is the degree of independence in practical matters (such as washing, dressing, going to the toilet, going shopping alone) which is both possible for the child at his age and allowed or encouraged by his mother. On the other, there is the degree of emotional dependence displayed by the child, which may be in accordance with what the mother thinks desirable or not. The child may resist his mother's attempts to modify his behaviour, so that in spite of her best efforts he may continue to be more or less independent than she would like in either or both of these respects. When handicap imposes a degree of physical dependence quite inappropriate to the age of the child, the issue is further complicated for the mother, the child and anyone who attempts to make judgments about them.

For these reasons, a different approach to the problem was

[1] An interesting account of the difficulties of defining the 'normal' family and then of making contact with its members for research purposes, is given in *Family and Social Network* by Elizabeth Bott. Social Science Paperbacks, London, 1968.

[2] Wright, Beatrice A. *Physical Disability—a Psychological Approach.* Harper & Row, New York, 1960.

adopted at Nottingham. There was readily available a great deal of information about the lives of normal 4-year-old children and their families. The mothers of 700 4-year-olds had given detailed accounts of how they had brought up their children so far and of how they had dealt with specific aspects of their children's behaviour. These data provided a ready made comparison group.[1] It is true that the sample of cerebral palsied children included many who were chronologically well beyond 4 years old but varying degrees of physical and mental handicap meant that for many of them their developmental level was similar to that of much younger children. In addition, their lives were not following the patterns that impose a modicum of independence on normal children (whether this is welcomed by mother and child or not); for example, nearly two thirds (76 out of 125, or 61%) of the cerebral palsied children who were 5 years or older had not been able to start school and only 22 of them were going to a day-centre of some kind for as much as 5 days per week. It has been pointed out elsewhere[2] that pressures for independence are often brought seriously to bear by mothers only when school is imminent and that this spur to action may be absent when a child is more than minimally handicapped.

Given these considerations, a comparison of a sample of normal 4-year-olds with a sample of handicapped children ranging from 1 to 8 years is more appropriate than it might at first seem. We therefore decided to compare the responses of the two samples of mothers to questions about all appropriate areas of day-to-day living and behaviour. These areas divide roughly into two main categories—one includes the internal relations of the family with one another, the other includes the experiences of the various family members in the wider social context. In the first of these two categories we asked mothers about:

The child's demands for attention*
Frequency of temper tantrums and how these were dealt with*
Use of 'comforters' at bedtime*
Indulgence by parents at bedtime*

[1] Newson, J. & E., 1968.
[2] Newson, J. & E. 'Child Rearing in Socio-cultural Perspective' in *The Spastic School Child and the Outside World*. Spastics Society & Heinemann, London, 1966.

Other children's feelings of jealousy*
Methods of discipline*
Father participation*
Agreement of parents on questions of upbringing*
Self-criticism by mothers*

and in the second:

The child's contacts with other children and encouragement
    of aggressiveness*
Extent of outings
Holidays
Mothers' feelings of loneliness
Mothers' actual contacts with family and friends
Mothers' reactions to casual interest in the child in public
Use of baby-sitters*
Parents going out separately

For each aspect of behaviour marked * there was comparable data about the normal 4-year-olds. Wherever it made good sense to do so, exactly the same questions were used for the handicapped children as for the normal children, when the mothers were interviewed.

Before discussing these comparisons, it might be interesting to consider how mothers see their handicapped children in terms of temperament and of being easy to manage. We asked them whether the children were 'happy or miserable a lot of the time'. The majority of them (90%) thought of them as being happy most of the time—this does not mean that the children are never miserable at all but that mothers are prepared to tolerate justifiable upsets, particularly when they realize that the children are often rather bored with the limited range of activities and amusements open to them. They still think of the children as being mostly happy after making these allowances. And of course, some of the children reported as being happy at the time of interview had been much less contented earlier in their lives. Still others are happy enough in the day-time but cry a great deal during the night, but again mothers do not think of these children as more miserable than happy on balance. To be counted as 'miserable', a child has to be inconsolably 'grizzly', or even screaming, most of the time. Some children are very quiet and apathetic, but these children too, are usually assumed by their mothers to be as happy as they can be in the circumstances. Some illustrations follow:

Boy: 3 yrs.

He's usually so happy, you know. He isn't grizzly or anything. He just sits there looking at a book and smiling when you look at him. (And of the same child)—Oh, he cries in the night, he screams all night. Last night he slept well, he woke up at 5.0 o'clock in the morning and started to scream. He's usually screaming all night. There's nothing you can do.

Boy: 5 yrs.

He's as happy as . . . he wakes up singing. 'Course, I have days when he does have little tantrums, which is only natural, but most of the time he's just like this all the time—we don't know he's here.

Girl: 3 yrs. (pilot study)

She is normally a very happy little girl. As I say—we are getting to the stage when I think she needs an outlet, and there doesn't seem an awful lot you can do with one hand. I can think of lots of things with two, you know, a little girl could do.

Girl: 2 yrs.

It just depends how she feels. Some days she'll want me to nurse her and other days she'll sit hours, and I just keep going up to her and talk to her, and she'll smile and that's it. She wants you to talk to her—'cos I think they've got a terrible life—they're terribly lonely. I mean, they're left out a lot, I should say. When you talk to her, you know, you don't know how much she understands or what she's thinking. I mean, I don't think they've got any life, myself, not unless they ever learn to walk and help themselves a bit.

The majority of these 'happy' children were considered to be easy to manage by their mothers but 42 of them (26% of this group) were not—their mothers agreed that they 'objected' to having things done for them or simply were awkward to handle in a physical sense. In some cases the children simply wanted to do things for themselves and be independent. In others it meant real difficulty for the mothers when it came to bath time or dressing the child or mealtimes—or sometimes all these things (see Chapter 3). Seven of the 18 children seen as generally 'miserable' were also difficult to manage. Thus, 2 out of 3 (66%) of all the children were both 'happy' and easy to manage so that it might be expected that they would not require such a disproportionate amount of their mothers' time that the other children in the family would be deprived of their share.

This contention is to a large extent supported by the mothers' replies to direct questions about the amount of attention demanded by the children. Fifty-six (31%) either always followed their mother around everywhere (if they were mobile though not necessarily walking) or would want to be with her if they caught sight of her as she worked around the house. The rest (69%) did not seem to be particularly demanding of attention. Twenty of the children could not safely be left alone in a room while their mothers got on with their work elsewhere. Seven of these were simply children aged between 1 year and $3\frac{1}{2}$ years whom one would expect to need a good deal of supervision. Two of them were between $3\frac{1}{2}$ and 5 years old—a $3\frac{1}{2}$-year-old boy who often fell down and a mentally handicapped 4-year-old who was very mobile although not walking. The remaining 11 children in this group were over 5 years old. All except one had mental handicaps—the exception was another child who fell down frequently. The mentally handicapped child, if mobile, can pose some of the greatest management problems for his parents—six of the eleven older children who could not be left came into this category. Of the remaining five, one was blind, another could not be left even in her chair because it tipped easily, one fell frequently, one lived in a caravan so that someone was always with her anyway and the last was described by her mother as 'spoiled' and very demanding of attention. In contrast, physically handicapped children can often be left for periods of time that are reasonably useful from the mother's point of view, so long as they are secure in their prams, cots or special chairs. Sixty-one children could be left for varying periods in this way. Some of the least mobile could even be left lying on the floor in complete safety.

These factors should be borne in mind when considering the contents of Table 4.I. It may be of interest to know that of the 28 children aged 3 years 6 months to 4 years 11 months, there were 16 who could be treated very nearly as normal 4-year-olds. Of this 16, 4 (25%) could be left for periods of up to 1 hour while the majority (75%) could be left for longer than an hour.

TABLE 4.I

Attention needs

	Normal 4-yrs.-olds	$1-3\frac{5}{12}$ yrs. N=27	C.P. sample $3\frac{6}{12}-4\frac{11}{12}$ yrs. N=28	5+ yrs. N=125
Can't be left	—	26% (7)	7% (2)	9% (11)
Can be left for up to 60 minutes	52%	26% (7)	32% (9)	22% (28)
Can be left for longer than 60 mins.	48%	48% (13)	61% (17)	69% (86)
	100%	100% (27)	100% (28)	100% (125)

The problem of balancing the needs of various members of the family is not unique to these mothers. In any family with more than one child, the mother has to learn to divide her favours equally and as needed—this can be difficult[1] and rivalry and jealousy inevitably occur in some circumstances in spite of the mother's best efforts to prevent them. The mothers of the handicapped children were asked if they thought the other children in the family ever seemed jealous of the handicapped one (the question did not arise in 39 families where there were no other children or where these were infants). The mothers of the normal children were asked whether the 4-year-old child ever seemed jealous of his brothers or sisters. In both samples,[2] 33% of the mothers replied that there had been some jealousy.

When asked whether they made special efforts to ensure that the normal children should not feel left out, 29 of the 46 mothers in the East Midlands sample who had reported some jealousy said that they tried to make up for the extra attention needed by the spastic child by giving extra love whenever they could to the normal children (24 mothers) or by giving them extra little presents or treats (5 mothers). Thirteen of the 105 mothers who had *not* reported jealousy also did this as a preventive measure but for the majority of mothers the problem had not arisen or was not felt to be serious enough to warrant any action. But sometimes explaining different approaches to discipline could be a difficulty, particularly where a child was too handicapped

[1] See Newson, J. & E., 1968, p. 93, for a graphic description of the demands that can be made on a mother of several children.
[2] These figures for the normal children have not been published.

mentally to understand the principles of punishment. Another difficulty arose in some instances when people outside the family tended to favour the handicapped child, no doubt in a well-intentioned attempt to compensate him a little for being handicapped. Some of these situations are illustrated in the following comments:

Boy: 8 yrs.

Q.: Do you think you make allowances for him more than for the other children?)

I don't think so, and I try very very hard not to do, because it would be terribly easy to spoil a handicapped child. In fact, I think in some ways I'm p'raps more strict—I think the little one (non-handicapped), I think he's got away with more than what the other one has because with a handicapped child you seem to have to be *extra* firm with them.

Boy: 6 yrs.

(Q.: Do the other children ever seem jealous of him for the attention he gets?)

Well, no. I think it's up to the mother to make sure they don't feel they're left out. I think it's most essential that they have the right sort of treatment. I try to act as normal as possible with *her* and treat him as a different . . . She helps me with him a lot—she feeds him, she runs up and down stairs for a nappy, she'll wash his face occasionally, she'll wheel him.

Girl: 7 yrs.

I don't think she's jealous—she's only jealous at the time when Margaret keeps having new shoes. The only other time—oh, there's another thing I don't like. If Margaret's shopping for me she'll probably come with a bar of chocolate or something—I think people feel sorry for her. Well, when they're twins, I think people ought to say 'Share this with your twin sister'. Even my husband's sister, I've seen her give that child half a crown and say 'You keep it to yourself and don't share it with the rest.' Well, I think it's wrong.

Boy: 8 yrs.

This is a thing we had to find out by trial and error; We found out that (his brother) Ivan was getting awfully jealous and I never realized it. This was one thing we *did* talk over with Dr ——

(general practitioner). Ivan was a marvellous baby, he really was good, and he was a child who was perfectly clean by a year old: and after Adrian came out of hospital, Ivan would be about 3, and he started wetting the bed. I couldn't figure it out, I never tried to make him jealous. But he went on till he started school, till he was 5. The doctor explained that it was . . . He never *did* anything to Adrian. He never pinched him or hurt him in any way, never *showed* any jealousy but the doctor said that it was his way of getting attention. The jealousy was there. Then—Ivan would be about 6 and he'd been naughty and I gave him a jolly good thrashing and he turned round and said, 'Well, Adrian does it and you don't smack him.' As I say, it's one of those things that you don't realize and the doctor said to me, 'Well, there's nothing wrong with Adrian. He knows when he's being naughty, and if he's naughty, smack him.' And so I did. When he'd been naughty, then he got a smack and I found that Ivan was better as well; there was a better relationship between Ivan and Adrian. But I've still got to be a little bit careful.

Boy: 7 yrs.

She'll say, 'It's me you're shouting at again, not him. It's always me that does wrong, not him.' And yet if you shout at him or anything, she's upset. She thinks he shouldn't be shouted at . . . But in some ways I think she thinks he's like he is—somehow done to upset *her*—I don't know how to explain it. She's that sort of child, you know, she puts herself always in the wrong—everyone else is right and she's in the wrong.

Another mother had noticed a similar reaction:

Girl: 5 yrs.

Well, the teachers seem to think that he does (i.e. seem to be jealous), I think in the respect that he's got a chip on his shoulder—why should it have to be *his* sister and not anyone else's, you know.

To illustrate this question a little more, we asked mothers whether they had much trouble with the other children's behaviour in general, in order to discover how many of them were perhaps expressing their jealousy indirectly. In only eleven instances were mothers worried about the way the other children were behaving. The majority either thought their normal children were 'no trouble' or that they were only as much trouble as one might expect any children to be.

It may be of some relevance that in 8 out of the 11 families where the normal brothers or sisters were giving their mothers some anxiety, there were circumstances in addition to the presence of a handicapped child which could affect the other children. Five of these families had had some kind of disrupted fathering as well as a handicapped member—1 father had died, 3 were involved in considerable marital discord, 1 father was away from home for much of the time and was non-participant when present. In one family, the child worrying the mother was adopted and she thought it was this, not the handicapped brother that bothered him. In another, the mother had been told by the health visitor that her elder son was backward at school because the younger one was handicapped (a very naughty, active, hemiplegic child)—this mother had also had a baby die in infancy, when the older boy was 3 years old.

In only one instance did the mother relate the other children's behaviour to the handicap, and she described the older sister (6 years old, 4 years older than the handicapped child) as becoming upset and quiet when it became obvious that there was something wrong with the baby.

The question of disciplining the handicapped child was raised by a mother in one of the discussions about jealousy (see above). Mothers said many times in the course of the interview that they try to bring up their handicapped children in the same way as the normal children as much as they possibly can. Often they are advised to do so by doctors or other professional workers with whom they are brought into contact. But once again we must remind ourselves that we are talking about a very hetero-geneous group of children. The advice to 'treat him as a normal child' may be sensible for the lightly handicapped. For the parents of the severely handicapped and the mentally handi-capped, this advice may be quite unrealistic and actually worsen their dilemma—the dilemma of knowing on the one hand that they have a child who is anything but an ordinary child, whose differences they must accept, and to whom they must re-adjust their behaviour and expectations in many ways; yet at the same time of having to beware of favouring this child at the expense of the rest of the family, to avoid 'spoiling' him and teach him to become an acceptable member of society. The replies of the mother of a 5-year-old boy with moderately severe physical handicaps, and a hearing deficit which had affected his speech, express this very well. He was a very mobile child, although he could not walk. It was uncertain whether he had any intellectual impairment. He was a mischievous, lively boy who was included in the normal control patterns of the family. As he went to a special school, he spent the usual amount of time away from home and in the company of other children. His mother's answers to several questions are given below in the order in which they occurred.

> I think he needs *more* discipline than an ordinary child, because I think life's going to treat him a lot harder than it is a normal child and he's got to accept that fact . . . No, I try not to (make allowances for him and let him 'get away with things'). It's very difficult —I might be taking the wrong attitude about this, I don't know. But as I say, I think he's got to take a lot from life, so I try to school him *for* that, you know what I mean? It's just that life is going to be far more difficult for him so if I give him everything he wants it's going to be an awful shock when he goes out in the world and he's *not* getting everything . . . I think accepting the fact that they are different from normal children is half (the battle)—once you sort of accept that they *are* different—I mean, you don't believe it at first, at least, I didn't. I thought they'd made a mistake. And I do think that you don't—although you *try*—you don't quite see your own children as they are. I don't think you see *normal* children as other people see them. I think it's very hard to keep an unbiased opinion of them. I try not to spoil them. I think it's so easy to spoil these children . . . The physiotherapist (at hospital) said when he was one year old, 'Treat him as normal and belt him when he bloody well needs it!'

This mother made it quite plain that she was trying to prepare her child for what she thinks will be a hard life. She was not *quite* sure that she was doing the right thing and said that her husband was 'more chicken' about him than she was—she said he agreed with her in principal, but tended to 'backslide' when she was not there. The mother who speaks next also felt the need to train her 4-year-old girl to become the sort of person that other people would accept. The little girl was walking and able to get into as much trouble as most children, but her mother did not think she was as naughty as most children of her age. She was smacked most often for disobedience. Her father had views which were directly opposed to those of the mother.

Mother: I do let her go on and on until I think, Well, she's either got to have a smack or let her rule *me*—you know. Any child's got to have a smack now and again. It sounds as if I'm tapping all the time but I'm not. I don't hit her unless it's really necessary, but I don't think that because she's a spastic she should get away with it, if you understand what I mean. Because his Mam (husband's mother) was saying don't hit her, she can't help it. But if I don't bring her up for other people to like her, how can I expect other people to put up with it—you know . . . I don't like hitting her but I *have* to . . . I never smack her unless I'm really fed up with it. I can say—I like to talk to her—I say 'Come on, come on' and then perhaps I'll smack her but I don't smack her to hurt her. Her dad always says I do.

Father—later in interview: You can't *make* these children do anything—you've got to persuade them into it, you know.

Both the mothers quoted echo the general attitude found among the majority of mothers of normal children, that smacking simply cannot be avoided, although the reasons behind this attitude vary considerably.[1] Some mothers, for instance, are driven to it by their own feelings or moods more often than-not; they smack unwillingly because it 'relieves their feelings', not because it is really effective. Others believe so firmly in its effectiveness as a deterrent that they smack quite calmly and deliberately. It is also not uncommon to dislike smacking but at the same time to use it because it seems to work.[2]

The combination of mental handicap with a certain degree of mobility probably creates the most puzzling situation for mothers. The child is physically quite capable of doing things which would undoubtedly be considered naughty if he were normal. Does he, however, understand that he should not do them? Will he understand and profit from his mother's attempts to teach him what is permissible and what is not? The comments that follow are those of mothers whose children are mentally handicapped, with varying degrees of physical handicap.

Boy: 5 yrs. Very mobile in house

He's quite mischievous. He does things on purpose—he runs away from me and then turns round and laughs if I tell him to come to

[1] Newson, J. & E. op. cit. Chapter 13.
[2] Newson, J. & E. op. cit. Chapter 13. 'Whether smacking is in fact effective as a long term socializing measure is a judgment which we cannot make at this stage.

me sometimes. He's like a baby, really. If I leave him long enough he'll empty all the cupboards, take all the pots out of the kitchen and that kind of thing. He does what babies do, only with him being so big, he's done them in half the time. (Do you think smacking does any good?) Yes, smacking his hand does because he knows not to touch things. But if I get angry and shout at him and smack, I frighten him and he just screams. By the time he's finished screaming, he forgets what it's all about and is just bewildered.

Boy: 6 yrs. Limited mobility but can use hands

There's nothing I can do when he's naughty. Sometimes when the food's on the table and I've been called away, I move the chair as far away as possible but he'll often manage to get to the table, get it off and it will drop on the floor with a terrific crash and he thinks it's a huge joke, the noise of the crockery. You feel you can't do anything because he doesn't understand.

Boy: 6 yrs. Very restricted mobility

Father: He gets his backside warmed up for him.
Mother: Sometimes afterwards I wonder if it *is* any good, really. I just really smack his hand, just to see. Like a normal child—you smack their hand—they know that they've got a slap because they've been naughty and they won't have to do that again. But the other day I smacked his hand—I was looking at a book and he wanted it and I said 'Don't do that' and smacked his hand. It were quite hard and he just looked at it and he *almost* cried. And that's the first time he's ever done it. And afterwards I felt sorry that I'd done it, you see, because he *doesn't* cry and I felt I shouldn't have done it. But I think *that's* a mistake because I think if you do hit a child you shouldn't 'love' it afterwards, because they can get the boss of you.

Later this mother said that her son could not understand any of the other sorts of control, such as putting him to bed or depriving him of sweets but that she would use these if he were normal or if she had any normal children. She went on to say:

Probably I would smack him, too, because I think it's the natural thing to do. I don't believe in *not* smacking children—like, some people believe in bringing children up psychologically, don't they, and I've known children that have developed into real rebels that have been brought up psychologically. And *we* used to get smacked and my husband too, and I don't think we're delinquents. We didn't like it at the time. No child *likes* being smacked; but we don't hate our parents because they smacked us. I know him so well—I think he isn't naughty on purpose. If he does do things he's not aware that he's been naughty. He's such a good boy, he doesn't really do naughty things.

This last mother is obviously trying to think through the situation in terms of what she feels is the right thing to do with a normal child. As she is not sure how much her child can understand (he was not talking at the time of interview) she has no idea how to modify her attitudes to smacking or even if she should modify them at all.

The next three mothers, in contrast, are quite sure how they should proceed, two of them because they are sure that smacking is inappropriate to a child who cannot understand right from wrong (they are also quite sure their children really cannot understand) and one because she is against smacking in principle.

Girl: 2 yrs. Very mobile. Appears to make no response either to her environment or to people

We never smack her because she's never needed smacking. She doesn't even know if she is doing something she shouldn't. She doesn't know, you see—at least *I* don't think that she knows. Not like with some children—I have a little girl comes in here and she's a wee bit younger than Michele, but of course she knows that she shouldn't touch everything in people's houses, but she still does do, and I feel to myself that this little girl should be smacked, you see. Because she does know that she shouldn't have these things. But, you see, it's no use saying No to Michele, because she doesn't know what No means.

Girl: 5 yrs. Not mobile

Oh, I smack the others but they know right from wrong. They understand. I've never smacked her . . . Mind you, I can understand people—you can get to the pitch . . . I've shouted, I've often shouted 'Oh, for goodness sake shut up, child.' But it's never crossed my mind to smack her. It's never entered my head. My husband and I have had words but I think that's the way you relieve your feelings—you relieve them with each other, more so than on the child because you know the child can't help it. Because even if you smacked them, you wouldn't help *them*. They wouldn't know—well, she wouldn't know, anyway.

Boy: 18 mths. Not mobile (pilot study)

No, I don't think it necessary to smack most children. No, I think they can be chastised in other ways—not *him*, but such as (his sisters), anybody all right . . . No, there's no need to smack. But there again, I've never been hit in my life so therefore it doesn't appeal to me to start knocking these about.

All the children we have talked about in this context have been able to behave in such a way that they evoke responses in their mothers which could lead to smacking, for one reason or another. Even the little girl of 5, quoted last but one, had quite frequent spells of screaming that her mother found hard to bear, although her response was to shout not to smack. There are, however, a few cerebral palsied children who are both severely mentally and physically handicapped and who, at the same time, seem to be so little aware of their surroundings that nothing upsets them. These children do not have even occasional screaming spells. One mother said that caring for such a child was 'just like look-ing after a living doll'. There can be no question of smacking such a child either as a punishment or as a method of training him. He cannot even drive his mother to the point of smacking in exasperation. This must be one of the most baffling and least rewarding situations for a mother. One who had a child of this kind, a child who gave no sign that he knew whether she was there or not, had tried giving him a little slap 'in fun, you know, to make him cry or shout' but this was in no sense a punish-ment, merely an attempt to make her child acknowledge her existence.

These examples will help to remind us that mothers have different ways of approaching the question of the social training of their children, and that they are attempting to put their philosophies into practice in widely differing situations. Some indication as to the degree to which it is possible to 'treat them as normal', is provided by mothers' responses to questions about how they controlled their children's behaviour. Whenever it made good sense to do so, the East Midlands mothers were asked the same questions about their methods of discipline as were the mothers of the normal 4-year-olds. All of them were asked about smacking, but there were some instances when the questions about other methods of discipline were plainly in-appropriate, because the child was so young or so severely physically and/or mentally handicapped. The interviewer had to use her discretion over using or omitting these questions.

Mothers were first asked what their views were on smacking in general. In both samples, the majority of them approved of smacking in principle—8% of the East Midlands and 17% of the Nottingham mothers expressed disapproval of this practice. One hundred and four (71%) of the East Midlands group who had other children said that their policy on smacking was the same for all the children in the family, but 42 of them felt that smacking was not appropriate for the handicapped children, either because their mental handicap prevented their understanding what it meant, or because they were too young or too handicapped to be naughty in the same sense as ordinary children.

But of course smacking is not the only way in which mothers attempt to control their children, and some mothers who did not smack their handicapped children used other ways of showing their displeasure with naughtiness. Their replies were once more compared with those of the mothers of the 4-year-olds (see Tables 4.II and 4.III).

Only 9 children (5%) of the whole sample were exempted from all discipline. Seven of these 9 children were severely physically

TABLE 4.II

	Smacking	
	Normal 4-year-olds N = 700	East Midlands Spastics N = 180
Mother smacks:		
Only in anger	51%	35%
Only when calm	21%	22%
Both	25%	10%
Never or almost never	3%	33%
	100%	100%
Excludes spastic child because of handicap (N = 146)[1]	—	29%
No difference between spastic child and normal sibs.	—	71%
		100%

[1] These are families with more than one child.

TABLE 4.III

Other methods of discipline

Method	Normal 4-year-olds N = 700	East Midlands C.P. Sample	
Sent to bed	36%	30%	
Deprived of sweets, etc.	69%	38%	N = 142
'I won't love you'	36%	25%	
'I'll send you away/ leave you'	27% (N = 422)	23%	N = 85*
Threaten with authority figure	27%	27%	N = 152

* For both samples, this question was *always omitted* if the child was present.

handicapped and had been included in our 'uncertain' category as to mental status: the other two were known to be very mentally retarded. It may well be that the concepts of naughtiness and of punishment really are inappropriate to such children, and that mothers are realistically recognizing this fact when they exclude them from the normal forms of control. However, it is obvious that most mothers attempt to use the methods that they find suitable for their particular children in 95% of this sample. Most of the children who were not smacked were disciplined in other ways, and similarly most of those who were exempted from some or all of the other forms of punishment were smacked. When mothers said that they did not use some of the forms of control other than smacking, they were asked if they would do so if the child were not handicapped—51% of the whole sample said that they were making no distinctions because of the handicap. Of the remaining 49%, about half (25% of the whole sample) were making exceptions because of the handicap, and the other half had not been asked the questions because the interviewer had decided to omit them.

It seems from this evidence that most mothers include their handicapped children in the family patterns of control as much as they can, but they do have to modify their approach to this area of child-rearing where the degree or kind of handicap dictates. In particular, the use of methods of discipline other than the immediate smack entails a level of conceptual understanding beyond the capacity of severely mentally retarded children, and for the severely physically handicapped most forms of naughtiness and mischief are out of the question. In addition, when children already have severe limitations on their pleasures, mothers are understandably reluctant to deprive them further. But this necessary difference of approach to the problem of control does not always breed resentment in the normal brothers and sisters. One mother said, 'They think she ought never to be smacked or anything like that. Oh yes, if I smack her, they go mad. They love her,' but another *had* found this a source of difficulty—'He never does as he's told because he doesn't know what it is. It's very difficult to discipline the other children because of it, actually, because they say "Oh, well, *he* does this, *he* wets his nappy." You know, that's the main difficulty.' Both points of view were echoed by others, for example on pp. 85 and 86 of this chapter where mothers are talking about possible causes of jealousy among the other children in the family. Mothers have to try to explain to the brothers and sisters why more is expected of them than of the handicapped child, even though the cerebral palsied one may be older. Discussing the problem of the 4-year-old who was expected to go to the toilet although her 7-year-old sister was not, one had this to say:

> I used to think, well, have I to smack Cathy to go to the toilet, and yet you couldn't smack Teresa, 'cos there was no point in it. Cathy—she still says it—'I can go to toilet because I *can* go to toilet. Teresa doesn't go because she *can't* go to toilet.' I mean, you've got to talk to your others to make 'em understand. (Interviewer: Do they understand that you have to make allowances for her, or do they think she gets away with things and this isn't fair?) Well, they've never said anything . . . I tell them she's not like them but she really has to be loved like a baby. There's nothing else you can say to them. They wondered, you know, why she wasn't going to their school and that. I said 'Oh, she's going to this school (training centre) to learn to talk and run about with them, and as soon as she's ready, she'll be off to your school,' and they accept that. You know, just tell 'em she was born small . . .

Mentally handicapped children also go on behaving in ways which although acceptable in babies and very young children, are actively discouraged in older normal children. In this situation, the mother has to decide whether to treat all her children alike and risk punishing the handicapped child for something which he cannot understand is wrong, or whether to discriminate between them and risk offending the normal child. The mother

who speaks next had already met this problem and was antici-
pating more trouble of the same kind in the future. The child
with cerebral palsy was 6 years old and her sister 4 years.

> Now, once Katie (4) went through a habit of biting. Well, Chris-
> tina bites if she gets the chance—a couple of times Katie's been
> cuddling her and she's bit her (Katie's) face. Well, I don't smack
> Christina for it, but Katie went through a phase of biting and she
> bit Christina a couple of times on her arm and she got a smack
> for it. And she did say to me then, 'Well, Christina bites.' I had
> to say to her 'Well, Christina's too little to understand yet.' You
> know, it's very difficult. I think that is going to be a big problem,
> trying to explain.

It is not difficult to think of whole areas of activity where a
similar problem could arise, even if children with physical
handicaps were mentally normal. At the table, for example, a
child with poor hand control might often drop cups and spill
food, for which he could not in fairness be chastised although
his brothers and sisters might be. Probably only the mother
herself can decide how much social training of this kind is
appropriate for her particular child. She then has to convince
the other children of the justice of her decisions and also to
reconcile these decisions with her avowed intention to 'treat
him as normal' as far as she can. The last mother quoted above
said later, 'I do try to treat Christina as much normal as I
possibly can. I sort of treat her more as I probably would a
baby. I don't try to make *more* of Christina than Katie.'

Just over half the mothers (93) said that they had to make some
allowances for their children and that they expected less of them
than of the normal children in the family, even when the latter
were younger than the handicapped child. Only 12 (13%) of
these thought that any of the other children actually resented
this necessary discrimination, although most had taken trouble
to explain to the others why it was necessary in order to forestall
resentment. Where there was a considerable age gap between
the handicapped child and the older brothers and sisters, it was
naturally much easier for them to accept that he had to be
treated differently. It was often commented that they spoiled
him into the bargain. Very young or infant brothers and sisters
also presented no problems. Even when children were fairly
close in age, the resentment was not always that the handicapped

one was not *disciplined* as the others were. A 4-year-old, for example, found it hard to see why he should struggle to dress himself when his 6-year-old sister was still dressed and fed like a baby. His resentment was part of a pattern found to be common among the Nottingham sample of 4-year-olds—loss of interest in the acquisition of a skill which has been a challenge at 3 but becomes a bore at 4.[1] To have an older sister who is still being relieved of this chore makes it all the harder to bear.

However, although resentment on the part of brothers and sisters did not seem to be a major problem to the mothers in the East Midlands sample, this may be a situation that changes as the family grows up. Adolescents may find the restrictions of having a child around who is developmentally much younger than his years more irksome than they did when they were all younger. For example, one mother said that the older children resented having their evening viewing of television interrupted by the shouting of the handicapped child, who could not understand that he was required to keep quiet at this time. Another 11-year-old sister resented the restrictions on outings imposed by her handicapped brother's need to be taken everywhere in a wheelchair which would not fold for travelling (the family had no car). This same girl, however, was 'ever so good with him, she's sat there all day while I've been washing and read to him' —a reminder that the other children's feelings are more likely to be mixed than to consist entirely of tolerance or resentment.

Temper tantrums are another aspect of children's behaviour which is bound to call forth some sort of response on the part of the parents both of the normal and the handicapped. Tantrums were by no means rare among the normal 4-year-olds—only 32% of them were reported as never having any at all and the same was true of the spastic children (31%). However, there was a difference between the two samples as to the frequency of tantrums—daily and almost daily occurrence was reported more than twice as often for the total handicapped group as for the normal group, 22% and 9% respectively. This difference is great enough to have statistical significance[2] and it holds for all the spastic children aged 3 years and over. (The 8-year-olds in the sample are the exception—35% of these had daily tantrums but there is no clear indication as to why this should be so.)

[1] Newson, J. & E., op. cit., 1968.
[2] $\chi^2 = 20 \cdot 9$ $\eta = 1$ $P < \cdot 001$.

When a difference as great as this occurs, it is necessary to look for an explanation. In this case, there seem to be two important contributory factors which are themselves inter-related. The first of these factors is that a high proportion of the handicapped children having daily tantrums were unable to talk at all or had serious difficulties in communication—higher, that is, than one would expect if speech were of no importance here.[1] This means that they were deprived both of a way of expressing feelings of anger or frustration and of a means of avoiding frustration. By the time normal children are 4 years old, verbal communication is of paramount importance to both mothers and children. Not only can mothers reason with their 4-year-olds and issue quite complex verbal instructions in the confident expectation that they will be understood, the child also by now has a powerful weapon with which to resist her control—the well-known phenomenon of 'answering back'. This, combined with 'cheek', provides outlets for defiance and self-assertion which are denied to the child who cannot talk. In addition, such a child cannot let his mother know whether he is hungry, in pain, bored, tired or longing for company—he cannot tell her how he feels about anything. In this situation, it must be inevitable that much is done to him that he does not want and just as much left undone that he does want. This brings us to the second factor which contributes to the high incidence of temper tantrums in the handicapped group.

For the normal group of children it was quite clear that both mothers and researchers attached similar meaning to the term tantrum. 'The temper tantrum is the child's response to extreme subjective frustration: that is to say, the child appears to think that he is being severely frustrated but children differ con-siderably as to what objective event triggers off this behaviour. Exaggerated aggression is shown, though not necessarily against the mother unless she gets in the way of it: indeed, it is charac-teristic of the temper tantrum that aggression is rather general-ized in its expression, directed against the environment as a whole, and sometimes also against the child himself. It is also typical that the tantrum is an emphatic statement to the world at large of the child's anger, rather than having any effective

---

[1] $\chi^2 = 3.74$ $\eta = 1$ $p < 0.6$. This is very close to significance at the 5% level. 27% of the children without speech had daily temper tantrums—almost twice as many as of those with speech, where the proportion was 14%.

function in putting right what has frustrated him.'[1] A close look at the actual behaviour which counted as tantrums in the handicapped group, related to the degree and kind of handicap of the individual children concerned, reveals that although this definition is adequate for some of them, mothers had also included in this category, behaviour which could more plausibly be interpreted in other ways. For example, a mentally handicapped boy of 6, at home all day without companions, who could roll around the floor but not sit up, who could not talk and who appeared to understand only a little of what was said to him, who had no interest in toys or anything else, had daily screaming bouts that his mother called temper tantrums. In fact, such a boy can really provide no clues whatsoever about the real meaning of his screaming. When his mother was asked what she thought it was that started it, she suggested that it might be boredom or a desire to attract her attention. When she gave him her attention, however, and tried to sooth him, she was often unsuccessful, so much so that she was going to ask the consultant's advice about what to do when she next saw him.

Another mother of a 6-year-old girl equally severely handicapped, when asked, 'Does she ever have a real temper tantrum?' replied, 'Oh yes, in that way she's a completely normal child.' But in addition to her other handicaps there was a doubt as to whether this little girl's hearing was impaired. She could not talk but appeared to take an interest in her environment. She loved music, going for 'walks' in her chair and playing with empty boxes. In other words, she was capable of a degree of response to people and situations. As she, too, was having no day-care, and having no brothers or sisters, had to rely on the adults in the household for company and attention, her apparent tantrums could more easily be explained as attempts to impinge on her environment in the only way open to her, and to interact with the people around her.

A very active mentally handicapped boy who could not speak, screamed whenever he was required to do something he did not want to do. For example, he always refused to walk out in the street with his parents, although he walked in the house perfectly well. His mother could not guess why and he could not explain, but it seems more likely that his screams meant that he was afraid of something than that they were an expression of

[1] Newson, J. & E., op. cit., 1968.

generalized aggression caused by frustration. His temper was not ineffective, either, because he was getting his point across sufficiently well for his mother to give up attempts to make him walk to the shops. She took him in a wheelchair.

Other examples could be quoted, but these are sufficient to illustrate the point that whereas the mothers of the normal children are using the term temper tantrum to refer to a specific feeling on the part of the child, which he can express in a number of ways (i.e. verbally, by slamming doors, kicking, biting, by removing himself or by throwing himself to the ground and abandoning himself to his rage) the situation is reversed for many of the handicapped children. They have very limited forms of expression for what may well be a variety of emotions. Without speech or movement, or both, they can only scream whatever the cause of their distress. Mothers describe this as temper because this is the normal behaviour it most closely resembles.

Mental handicap may also have some bearing on this matter. When we look at the children aged 5 years[1] and over, we find that 29% of all those with confirmed mental defects had daily or almost daily tantrums. This is 3 times as large as the proportion of 5+ children who had been classified as having normal intelligence—9% of these had daily or almost daily tantrums. Degree of physical handicap did not seem to be similarly related to tantrums—22% of the mildly physically handicapped had daily tantrums and so did 17% of the severely physically handicapped.

There were 40 children in the East Midlands sample having temper tantrums most days. Eighteen of these children had normal speech or little difficulty with communication. They were also mobile and were able to exhibit behaviour which came close to the normal child's expression of temper. However, half of these 18 children had some degree of mental handicap. If these are left out of consideration, the remaining 'nearest to normal' children having daily or almost daily tantrums amount to 5% of the sample.

Mothers of the handicapped children sometimes said how distressing it could be when the child screamed and screamed and could not be comforted. There were differences between the

[1] Five years is taken as a cut-off point because children are more likely to have been 'ascertained' as mentally handicapped at this age than the younger children.

replies of the two groups to questions about how they dealt with tantrums. Whereas 33% of mothers of normal 4-year-olds resorted to smacking, 23% of the East Midlands mothers did so. Twenty-one per cent with normal children used love, sympathy and/or distraction as opposed to punishment and so did 34% of the East Midlands mothers. This difference in approach may be related to the mental handicaps of some of the cerebral palsied children. Just as mothers are reluctant to punish children who cannot understand the concept of naughtiness, they feel that it is not right to punish them for having tantrums if they cannot help having them, for one reason or another. Some think tantrums may be an expression of the frustration imposed by handicap and are prepared to tolerate them for this reason, although this does not make them any easier to cope with. Many of the mothers faced with this situation, said they were really puzzled as to what to do for the best, and would have been very relieved if someone could have told them categorically that it would be best either to smack or not, and if not, what else they could do. In the quotation that follows, the mother of a 3-year-old girl, seen at the pilot stage of the study, expresses this kind of uncertainty.

> She was really going mad—sort of hitting me and half stroking me because she couldn't decide whether she loathed me or not and I thought 'Well, it's no good trying to tell her to control herself, better get it out. So I laid her on my lap and said 'Hit me.' I thought it would be a good thing. Do you think it would be a good idea to smack them? Is this an age for having tantrums? Why is that? Is it frustration—partially? Because she hasn't got an outlet, has she? I asked (the physiotherapist) and she said she didn't think she could help me. She didn't know quite *what* to say!

There was a feeling among the mothers of the normal children that they ought to be able to teach their children to control their temper and, moreover, that if they did not succeed in doing so they (the mothers) would be open to criticism from such people as teachers, doctors and nurses.[1] We have already suggested that the need to prepare their children for school life may be a spur to mothers of normal children in their efforts to encourage independence. The same need may also contribute to their greater readiness to punish their children for tantrums—in the

[1] Newson, J. & E., 1968.

hope that they may learn more quickly by this means that
'temper' is not acceptable behaviour. When a child is handicapped and is in obvious ways like a child much younger than
his years, it is difficult for the mother to decide what sort of
behaviour it is reasonable to expect from him. In addition, she
does not always have the imminence of school to reinforce
whatever convictions she may hold about the need to encourage
the control of temper.

The mothers in the East Midlands sample who had asked
doctors' or other professional advice had met either bewilder-
ment equal to their own, advice to smack or advice not to
'give in' to the children—this last an echo of the attitude of
some mothers themselves that their children are small adver-
saries in some kind of contest. One mother of a handicapped
girl 2½ years old, who smacked her daughter for tantrums, said,
of smacking in general, 'I think you have to show 'em who's
boss—I smack *him* (brother) and he's only 10 months.' When
asked what kind of naughtiness she would smack for, she
replied 'If she's on—you know—and she don't seem to know
what she's on *for*. If she's roaring and that. And sometimes you
get two on 'em—and *he's* on and *she's* on and you don't know
whether you're coming or going, you know. *You've* got children, haven't you? Well, you know, then—I don't think a man
understands.' The next mother describes how she tries to avoid
being forced into smacking:

Girl: 6 yrs.

She does get upset and when she does I can't do anything with her
at all but I can never find out why. It never seems to be anything
particularly that triggers it off—you know—she just seems as if
she'll be sitting there one minute, then she'll start to cry and I
think, oh perhaps she's thirsty and I give her a drink, but she
doesn't want that and once she starts, it keeps going on and she
cries and she screams, and I just can't do anything with her at all,
when she's like that. (Interviewer: What *do* you do?) Well, if I
can't—if cuddling her and giving her a drink and changing her
nappy does nothing for her, I usually go and lay her down on the
bed and I just let her cry because I must admit that I find when
she's in one of these moods I can't cope with it. I feel as though I'm
going to shake her, you know, to sort of stop her, so I think, well,
rather than hit her for it, because, I mean, she doesn't understand
what she's doing, you see, so I don't hit her for it, so I think, Well,

if I don't put her in the bedroom out of the way, I *am* going to hit her. So I put her in the bedroom and I just let her cry it off. She gradually cries it off and usually ends up going to sleep after it and then I get her up and give her a drink.

The mother quoted next was one of those who did not punish her child for temper tantrums. Instead, she sometimes put her in her cot until she had got over it. The kind of explanation she had been offered may have had something to do with her greater tolerance of this kind of behaviour in the handicapped child— she said during the interview that similar behaviour in her normal little boy upset her far more.

Girl: 7 yrs.

Well, the doctors at London said—you know, like, the assessment at London—they explained it a bit more—the doctor there was quite good, really. He said that she would have these temper tantrums, she would have them instead of fits, you know, it cured the fits but it left her with those instead. And it's not so bad in a way as keep having fits but it's just that it upsets the whole house when she starts screaming and carrying on.

This topic has been discussed at some length because it seemed to be one which was more complicated for the mothers of the handicapped than the normal children. Because of the added difficulties, the possibility arises that questions of discipline and of upbringing in general might be a source of greater disagreement between their parents than it is for the parents of normal children. Mothers of the normal 4-year-olds were asked whether they ever felt doubtful that they were bringing up their children the right way, and whether they thought their husbands were more strict than they were. The East Midlands mothers were asked the same questions and also whether they and their husbands were in general agreement on questions of upbringing. Seventy-two (40%) of the East Midlands mothers sometimes wondered whether they were doing the right thing with their children as compared with 54% of the mothers of normal children. In view of the added difficulties of raising children who have handicaps, it could be argued that the difference might have been expected to occur in the other direction. On the other hand, as we have seen, there are fewer ways of controlling the handicapped children which are both acceptable to the mother and practicable than is the case with the normal children, so that there are fewer options about which to feel doubtful. In addition, about a quarter of the sample had been considered by the interviewer to be too handicapped for the question of being naughty to arise and almost another quarter were partially exempted from disciplinary measures by their mothers because of their handicaps. These factors may account both for the smaller proportion of self-critical mothers and for the smaller proportion of fathers who were considered by their wives to be stricter than themselves—21% (38) of the East Midlands sample, as opposed to 39% of the normal 4-year-olds sample. Although questions were not asked about the feelings of the fathers towards their handicapped children, it was not unusual for mothers to mention this at one point or another in the interview, and some of them considered that their husbands had found it harder than they had themselves to overcome their grief at having such a child. One mother who was seen at the pilot stage of the project put the point very well:

> Having a handicapped child, you are handicapped yourself, you do feel handicapped—but I think my husband more so than myself, because he misses the things that a normal child, a boy, does. I mean, I don't want to boast or anything, but I have conditioned myself because I think if I had let myself go it would have been worse for my husband and the boy, you see. I've tried to be sensible about these things.

There was a higher degree of agreement between parents of the handicapped children on the question of strict enforcement of discipline than there was in the normal sample—47% and 37% respectively of mothers reporting agreement. Again, in view of the difficulties discussed above, it would not have been surprising to find a difference in the other direction. The reduction of opportunities to be naughty in the case of the handicapped children may be a factor here and so may the 'tender' attitude of fathers towards their severely handicapped children. Whatever the reason, there seems to be less dissension over the handicapped children than there is over the normal children, and there is some evidence to suggest that this is related in some way to the degree or kind of handicap. If all the children with severe physical handicaps, and all the children with any degree of confirmed mental handicap are removed from the East Midland sample, 74 children remain who are most closely comparable

with normal children (row 3 in Table 4.IV). The figures relevant
to this group on parental agreement over discipline more closely
resemble those for the normal 4-year-olds. Reference to rows
4 and 5 of the same table shows that agreement is highest where
the children have some degree of mental handicap, and that
husbands are considered to be least strict where there are severe
physical handicaps.

TABLE 4.IV

Husband and wife agreement on discipline

	Husband stricter	Wife stricter	Agreement
1. Normal 4-year-olds	39%	24%	37%
2. Total C.P. sample	21%	32%	47%
3. C.P. children with mild to moderate physical handicaps and without confirmed mental handicaps, $N = 74$	30%	35%	35%
4. C.P. children with confirmed mental handicap of any degree $N = 77$	17%	25%	58%
5. C.P. children with severe physical handicaps but without confirmed mental handicaps, $N = 29$	10%	42%	48%

When we asked the East Midlands mothers whether they
agreed with their husbands about most things connected with
bringing up the handicapped child, not only discipline, 67%
reported agreement. (There were no comparable general questions asked of the normal sample). Among those who reported
disagreement were some who said that they did not agree with
their husbands about anything, and some who differed only
about the question of whether the handicapped child should go
away to school or to residential care at some time, a problem
which does not arise for most parents of normal children.
Among the parents who generally agreed there were some who
did so only because the fathers were said by the mothers to
'leave all that to me'. Although it was evident that there was
considerable disharmony in a few families, there was nothing to
suggest that having a handicapped child made this more likely,
and the replies discussed above suggest the contrary. There is a
possibility that the most disruptive children or the children born

into families least able to meet the situation of having a handicapped member had already been taken into residential care of some kind and so were missing from the East Midlands sample. In tracing the East Midlands sample from the files available to us, we found that 31 children were away from home who would have otherwise been eligible for inclusion, 17 of them in permanent residential care and 14 at boarding schools. It is likely that there were others of whom we were not aware. If family difficulties are an important factor in the selection of children for residential care, it could account to some extent both for the low incidence of discord in the families in the East Midlands sample and also for the much more distressing situation described by Maureen Oswin[1] from her experience of children in a hospital school, experience which led her to say, 'The incidence of breakdowns and emotional stress amongst the parents of cerebral palsied children is possibly fairly high. Among 26 of the children whose families I had knowledge of, there were 5 cases of mental breakdown in one or other of the parents; 5 of the families could not manage their child at home; 8 of the marriages were broken; one child had no parents at all, being a foundling child.' Miss Oswin goes on to say, 'It is questionable, of course, whether the breakdown and emotional stress amongst the parents mentioned above were caused directly by worry over the handicapped child, or whether there was a potential liability in the parent to break down anyway.' If, for the sake of argument, we were to assume that all the 31 children we knew to be away from home came from families where they were the cause of dissension between their parents, the proportion of parents in agreement about their children would still be similar to that in the normal sample—41% of the spastics and 37% of the normal 4-year-olds. Almost a third (31%) of the parents of the children in the hospital school were separated or divorced as opposed to 2% of the East Midlands sample, but again, if we were to suppose that all the 31 handicapped children away from home, and so out of the sample, had had parents who were separated or divorced (which is highly unlikely) the divorce rate would still only be half that for the institutionalized children —16% as opposed to 31%. These are, of course, mere speculations but the possibility that generalizations made from small

[1] Oswin, M. *Behaviour Problems Amongst Children with Cerebral Palsy.* John Wright & Sons Ltd., Bristol, 1967.

groups of highly selected children are likely to err more on the side of pessimism than those made from the sample of children at home may err on the side of optimism, cannot be dismissed.

The fathers[1] of the East Midlands children were not only present in the majority of families—they were also sharing in the tasks of bringing up the children, handicapped and normal alike. Both groups of mothers were asked how often their husbands actually bathed, dressed and took care of their children, how often they read to them, played and sang with them and whether there was anything that they would *not* do for them. The replies for the normal 4-year-olds, the handicapped children and the brothers and sisters of the handicapped children were almost identical (see Table 4.V). Fathers in the East Midlands sample

TABLE 4.V

Father participation

	Normal four-year-olds N = 700	East Midlands Spastics N = 174*	East Midlands siblings N = 144*
Highly participant	51%	50%	49%
Fairly participant	40%	38%	39%
Non-participant	9%	12%	12%
	100%	100%	100%

* The figures are less than 180 because in some families there was no father and in others there were no siblings.

tended to have the same rating both for the handicapped child and for the normal children in the family. In some families there was a division of labour, with mother looking after the handicapped child or in some cases the youngest baby and father looking after the others. There was, however, no evidence to support the view that a high proportion of fathers of handicapped children are more involved with the children than would be 'culturally expected'[2] at least in the eyes of the mothers. Today's fathers expect to take a large share in the care of their

[1] There was no difference in the incidence of shift-working in the two samples; 30% of each sample worked shifts of some kind, some including night work, some consisting of permanent night work and some consisting of long or 'odd' hours and weekends. There was no evidence that fathers of handicapped children show a general tendency to alter their hours of working in order to spend more time with their handicapped children.
[2] Schaffer, H. R., op. cit.

children, in the Midlands if not in Scotland,[1] and in all social classes.

Finally, the question of how parents approach the business of getting their children to bed and to sleep remains to be discussed. This was an area of mother-child interaction where it seemed likely that mothers would be forced to 'baby' their children more than they would if they had not been handicapped and also one where there was evidence available from the normal 4-year-old sample.

It was expected that a large proportion of the handicapped children would be poor sleepers, difficult to get to sleep and waking often during the night. In fact, 71% of their mothers reported that they had no problems in getting their children to sleep, at the time of interview, although 24 of these children (13% of the whole sample) had had some difficulty in the past. Mothers were asked whether the children had to take any tablets or medicine at bedtime, and if so, what the tablets were, but although 12% of them had evening medication of some kind, it was not often clear whether this was specifically to induce sleep or was simply part of their anti-convulsant drug therapy or general sedation. In addition, some of the children having this kind of medication were not among those with sleeping problems, so that the replies to this question are not a good indicator of the incidence of such problems.

In the normal 4-year-old sample, 8% of mothers reported that they nursed their children, sat with them upstairs or maintained contact with them in some way until they fell asleep—described as the 'indulgent bed-time'. In the East Midlands sample, 11% of mothers reported similar behaviour and the difference is not great enough to have statistical significance. When it comes to waking up in the night, again there is no significant difference between the two groups—10% of the handicapped and 7% of the 4-year-olds waking up more often than not. Thirty-six per cent of the handicapped children never woke up at all and although the remaining 54% did sometimes wake up, they did not necessarily need attention.

Difficulty with sleeping then, seemed to be confined to a small proportion of the East Midlands sample. However, where it did occur it tended to persist after the age of 4—12 children aged 5 and over (10% of this age group) still needed their

[1] The work referred to was carried out in Glasgow.

indulgent bed-time, 25 aged 6 or over (26% of this age group) were still having trouble getting to sleep and/or waking during the night. Although numerically the problem may not be a major one, its importance to individual families should not be minimized. To have regularly disturbed sleep is very hard for parents to bear and can in some instances make a crucial difference to their ability to care for the child at home.[1]

Some parents meet the problem of giving children frequent attention during the night by having the child sleep in the same room as one or both of them. This was by no means unknown in the 4-year-old sample, but twice as many of the handicapped children shared the bedroom with one or both parents—28% as opposed to 13% of the 4-year-olds. Eighteen of these children were aged 4 or younger—included in this number were half the 1- and 2-year-olds, as one might expect,[2] and a quarter of the 3- and 4-year-olds. It is perhaps more surprising to find that the proportion of children aged 5 and older who are still sleeping in their parents' room is also 25%. However, before jumping to the conclusion that this fact has sinister implications, we should look at the circumstances which have contributed to it. These are, as one would expect, interrelated and in some families several factors operate.

First and foremost, in some homes there is such pressure on sleeping accommodation that it is unavoidable that one of the children must share the parents' bedroom. Most often this is because the house has only 2 or 3 bedrooms and there are several children, some of whom are of opposite sexes and have reached the age when they can no longer share a bedroom. It is usually the youngest and 'only' children who are chosen to stay with the parents.[3] In 17 instances in the East Midlands families, there was pressure on accommodation, either for the reason just given or for others—in 2 instances, for example, dampness in some of the rooms had made them unusable. Twelve of the 32 children concerned were literally the youngest in the family and another 8 were developmentally the youngest, regardless of their chronological age, because they were severely physically and mentally handicapped. Only 6 children did not have serious handicaps in this group, and when all factors were taken into consideration, in only 2 instances did there seem to be no reason

---

[1] See Chapter 3.   [2] Newson, J. & E., 1963, op. cit.
[3] Newson, J. & E., 1968, op. cit.

whatsoever for the child to continue to sleep in the parents' room.

When children do have disturbed nights it is practical to have them in the same room as the parents. They can be attended to without disturbing the other children in the family. Sometimes the parents decide that it is easier if the child sleeps with one of them so that the other may rest undisturbed. Five of the handicapped children slept in the same bed as one or both of their parents. This too, was not unknown in the 4-year-old sample. However, fewer of the mothers of the handicapped children said that they would take the children into bed with them if they woke up in the night, than of the 4-year-olds—40% as opposed to 66%. The difference may be explained partly by the number of older children in the East Midlands sample and partly by the fact that the normal 4-year-olds often invited *themselves* into the parents' bed, whereas the handicapped children were not always mobile enough to do this. The difference might have been expected to occur in the other direction if in fact parents of handicapped children exhibit a general tendency to 'baby' their children more than is necessary.

In addition to the comfort of the mother's own presence at bedtime—or perhaps in some instances because they are denied this[1]—some children turn to various comfort habits such as the sucking of dummies, bottles and pieces of fabric or the cuddling of a favourite soft toy. Sometimes the two sorts of 'comfort' are combined, as when children suck their thumbs at the same time as they are stroking a piece of blanket. The persistance of 'comfort habits' at bedtime among the sample of normal 4-year-olds was seen by the Newsons (op. cit.) as an expression of some children's need to find continuity and consistency in a world which seemed to them capricious and full of inexplicable events. Familiar toys and bedtime rituals provide an element of stability. Since many of the children in the East Midlands sample were functioning at a developmental level much lower than would have been expected of normal children of similar chronological age, it would not have been surprising to find a higher percentage of such habits among them than was found among the 4-year-olds. This was not the case, as the figures in Table 4.VI show.

[1] 68 of the handicapped children took a soft toy, cloth, bottle or dummy to bed with them. 13 of these also had "indulgent bed-times."

Physical handicaps could account for the difference to a certain extent—cerebral palsy sometimes means that children can suck only with difficulty or that it is not easy for them to get their thumbs into their mouths. On the other hand, as with seeking refuge in the parents' bed, it may have been that some of the handicapped children were unable to insist on the use of comforters in the same way as the normal children did. It was very plain from the replies of the mothers of the normal 4-year-

TABLE 4.VI

Use of 'Comforters' at bedtime

	Normal 4-year-olds N = 700	East Midlands Spastics N = 180
Dummy	14%	12% (10% 4-year-olds or under and 2% 5+)
Bottle	4%	1%
Thumb	16%	4%
Cloth	5%	less than 1%
Soft Toy	26%	24%

olds that they often merely co-operated, willingly or otherwise, in routines and habits which had been initiated by the children themselves. The relationship between mother and child is essentially an interaction process, with the mother receiving and acting upon cues supplied by the child in addition to her attempts to impose her own wishes upon him. For this reason, the possibility arises that severely handicapped children may be unable to supply appropriate cues, so that in some respects they may be missing some of the comfort they need. It has been suggested by one paediatrician that in this situation the mother should be helped to adjust her attitudes and actions towards the child 'before irreparable harm is done to the mother-child relationship'.[1] Simon Haskell,[2] speaking at a study group on cerebral palsy, went further and said, 'I hypothesize that all our C.P. children and adults are at risk psychiatrically because all through various critical phases of development, mechanisms which unite infant to mother instinctually are damaged. Moreover, if mothers are not reinforced by infants' responses in this reci-

[1] Wigglesworth, Dr Robert, in *The Practitioner*, No. 1150, Vol. 192, April, 1964. Contribution to a symposium on 'The Handicapped Child'.
[2] Haskell, Simon, in *Learning Problems of the Cerebrally Palsied*. Report of a Study Group held in Oxford, 1964. Published by The Spastics Society.

procal exchange, the grave risk that mothers' signals will be extinguished is ever present.'

To those who subscribe to views such as these, the evidence supplied by the mothers in the East Midlands should afford a measure of reassurance. These mothers, in describing how they meet the requirements of a group of children of various ages and degrees of handicap, demonstrate that, to a remarkable degree, their 'mothering' follows patterns similar to those employed by mothers who have only normal children. This should not really surprise us. Most of them are bringing up normal children and handicapped children at the same time. They have their experiences with their normal children to guide them. Where special difficulties arise with the handicapped children, they appear to adapt the procedures used with the normal children as common sense dictates. Even when the child is so handicapped that he can supply very little reward or 'feed-back', the great majority of mothers in the sample use their imagination to fill the gaps—the mothers of children who have no speech, for example, go on talking to the children in the hope of eventually gaining a response.[1] Where the handicapped child is the only one in the family, it is more difficult for the mothers to judge how to proceed and some of them mentioned this. But even in these circumstances, mothers are not operating in a vacuum. They bring cultural and social-class expectations to their role as mothers, and they have their own childhood experiences upon which to draw.

In particular, if young handicapped children and infants appear to have suffered because they have been deprived of essential stimuli normally supplied by the mother (as Haskell suggests in the paper quoted), this could be because of separation from the mother, not because the mother, though present, is failing to supply what the child needs. Almost half the East Midlands children had spent at least one period in hospital during their first year of life and for 45 of them (25% of the whole sample) this period had exceeded 30 days. Where this separation occurred because the babies were cared for initially in premature baby units, the essential mother-child interaction could not even begin until the child was several weeks old. In spite of these considerations, the mothers in the sample appeared to have overcome impediments to the establishment of relation-

---

[1] See quotation about a 2-year-old girl on p. 82 of this chapter.

ships with their children and, like the group of American parents of handicapped children studied by Ray H. Barsch,[1] 'They all seemed to have set about the business of rearing the handicapped child according to whatever set of beliefs they held about child-rearing in general, and few of them changed their basic set of beliefs, even in the face of difficulties encountered in their day-by-day practices.'

[1] Barsch, Ray H. *The Parent of the Handicapped Child.* Charles C. Thomas, Springfield, Illinois, 1968.

CHAPTER 5

FAMILY AND COMMUNITY

The family itself is an evolving social and cultural unit with a history, a life-style and a structure that preceded the entry of the damaged child into its midst. As the family moves through its life-cycle, its future course is moulded by the same variety of social forces that affect all families, as well as by the demands of the damaged child.

HOWARD R. KELMAN[1]

As we have seen, the internal patterns of family life seem to be disrupted less than one might expect by the presence of a young handicapped child. This may not continue to be so at adolescence, when both the handicapped and their normal brothers and sisters might find that the expected difficulties of this period of development are increased for them all. It would be most interesting and rewarding to see the same children again during their adolescence.

Turning now to the question of the family and its relations with the larger community, we have only two kinds of behaviour which can be directly compared with the sample of normal 4-year-olds.[2] The other topics on which there is information for the East Midlands sample were not relevant to the families of the normal children.

Taking first the idea that mothers of handicapped children—and indeed the other members of the family, too—will '*invariably* (our italics) go through feelings of isolation',[3] we asked the mothers in the East Midlands sample both whether they had experienced such feelings of loneliness and isolation and how much actual contact they had with relatives, friends and neighbours. We also asked how helpful people outside the immediate family had been and grouped the replies to all these

---

[1] Kelman, Howard R., op. cit.   [2] See Chapter 4, p. 81.
[3] Ibid, p. 76.

questions under three headings. The distribution of these replies is shown in Tables 5.I and 5.II.

TABLE 5.I

Loneliness and social contacts (a)

Amount of actual contact and support from relatives

Mothers' feelings	No relatives near	Very little	Adequate	Much support	Total	%
Lonely	2	9	18	9	38	21
Not lonely	4	13	74	51	142	79
Total	6	22	92	60	180	100

These figures show that 4 out of 5 mothers do not say that they feel any sense of isolation, and that the majority of the 21 % of them who *do* feel isolated are not in fact cut off from all social contacts.[1]

TABLE 5.II

Loneliness and social contacts (b)

Mothers' feelings	Amount of actual contact and support from friends				
	Very little	Adequate	Much support	Total	%
Lonely	10	19	9	38	21
Not lonely	22	77	43	142	79
Total	32	96	52	180	100

Similarly, some mothers who do not have a lot of contact with friends and relatives do not feel lonely in spite of this. It seemed that feelings of isolation were much more a function of the mother's personality than of the presence of a handicapped child. The comments of some of the mothers show this very clearly. However, the plight of mothers who *are* lonely and who *do* feel cut off, is very real. In particular, mothers in rural areas often experience practical obstacles to making the contacts they would like and having a child who is not easily transportable naturally adds to the difficulties. The mother speaking in the

[1] That the subjective experience of loneliness may not, for individuals, be accompanied by actual social isolation, is also shown by Peter Townsend in *The Family Life of Old People* (Routledge & Kegan Paul, London, 1957). He described the 'desolation' felt at the loss of a loved companion even when plenty of other companionship was available.

first quotation was in this situation and had two other young children as well as the eldest, who was severely handicapped. The second mother's actual situation was quite different—she lived in a small urban industrial area, had two children with six years between them and the younger was only mildly handicapped, yet she, too, had *felt* lonely, despite supportive friends and family.

Boy: 3 yrs.

Well, it is for me because I can't get out. The woman next door, well she's in her sixties and—you know—you've nothing to talk to her about and she doesn't often talk, she's all the time cleaning and that. Next door they go out to work and there's never anybody in. Of course, there's nobody around here, it's out in the country. I have never had anybody to talk to. I'm here for hours—well, *days*, sometimes, and never see anyone unless I go out in the car.

Girl: 5 yrs.

Yes, I do in some ways, because you're so busy looking after them that you haven't got time for going out . . . As I say, with her feeding she was very, very slow. Well, by the time she'd finished her feeding and that and I'd tidied round, it'd be time for her sister coming in at dinner-time—well, it was an effort to get out. I used to make myself go out on a Friday, to take her out in the pram and that. But I wouldn't like to go through it again, definitely not. I mean, it probably sounds a little bit selfish, saying you get no outside entertainment, but I think you need it and as I say, being on your own, you feel that nobody else has got this problem and you've got nobody to talk to about it. I mean, you tell your friends and that, and they pop in and see you but they don't understand the same—they *say* they do—they say, 'Oh, she'll be all right' but, I mean, even so, you've still got that loneliness.

Boy: 4 yrs.

Lonely? Well, no, quite the reverse, to be honest, because I find that people will stop and speak to you, you know.

Boy: 7 yrs.

Yes, I have done, but not now. I have found it, yes, when he was little. And I think if people helped you, if they would give you a kind word, I think it would help ever such a lot, from the mother's point of view.

Girl: 8 yrs.

It is true, people just don't want to bother with you—you can't do the same as they do, so they just don't bother with you.

Boy: 7 yrs.

Oh, *no*. Well, I think it just depends on how *they* (the mothers) are.

Girl: 5 yrs.

I wouldn't say I was lonely. I wouldn't say that sometimes I'm not *miserable*; I mean, I am, when I'm thinking about it—thinking how normal kids are, I do get (miserable)—not very often, I do have me moments. But I suppose—you haven't got one, have you? (Interviewer: No.) So you don't realize until it happens how heartbreaking it is.

Girl: 6 yrs.

Well, it depends if you've got any more in the family, really. If you've got others to attend to, like I have, well, you don't have time to *be* lonely.

Girl: 5 yrs.

Well, I admit I've got one or two children,[1] but there's times when I think to myself I should like to go out, even if it's only down to a friend's—or anywhere. I've always said as you can be lonely even when you've got a houseful of children. I know their daddies always say, 'Well, you've got the kiddies with you all day, how can you get lonely?' but I reckon you can, even when you've got children. I think if you only have a friend in half an hour a day, it makes the day go quicker. You have another *adult* you've spoken to, and that.

Boy: 7 yrs.

I shouldn't think so. I find being a housewife is a lonely job anyway as compared with going out to business.

Girl: 6 yrs.

We never mix. We mind our own business. They *would* help, you know—if I wanted to 'phone and there's anything wrong with her, but we don't bother asking for it. We've kept ourself to ourself.

[1] This mother had 10 children, all under 11 years old at the time of interview.

The support and comfort of friends and relatives who can 'drop in' can make all the difference to a mother with several young children who is tied to school hours and who finds taking out all the children together to visit people too much of a major operation—this is true even of families where all the children are normal but close together in age. The reality of such help was often made apparent during interviews when someone would come in for a cup of tea and a chat and finding a stranger present would slip out again with a promise to return later when it was convenient or with an offer to do the shopping as the mother was obviously tied up for the morning. The majority of mothers had this kind of contact with someone and some of the minority who did not would not have welcomed it— like the mother in the last quote, they 'kept themselves to themselves'. As one would expect, maternal grandmothers[1] living near by were often a tower of strength to their daughters and even when they lived far away were counted as supportive if they kept in constant touch, visited as often as possible and gave practical help such as making clothes for the handicapped child. Even at long distance, grandparents can convey general acceptance of the child and a sense of being on the side of the parents. Where this did not occur, mothers felt it very keenly, and a few even felt that they had to fight their own parents whose views on what was best for the child were contrary to their own.

However, accepting the interest, help and support of one's close friends and family is one thing. Facing the outside world and the curiosity of casual acquaintances or strangers is quite another. We asked the mothers how they felt about interest of this kind when they encountered people who did not know the children, on shopping or other expeditions. More than 70% of them said that they welcomed such interest, a fact which may be of interest to those who are hesitant to talk to them for fear of hurting their feelings. Genuine, sensible and non-advisory approaches are likely to be welcome. Tactless comment and gratuitous advice are not. Some mothers felt very strongly on this last point and had had some unpleasant experiences.

---

[1] So, of course, were many of the husbands' parents but it is more likely that a mother maintains close contact with her own mother after marriage. (See Young and Willmott, *Family and Kinship in East London*. Routledge & Kegan Paul, London, 1957.

Differing attitudes are expressed in the comments that follow:

Girl: 7 yrs.

Well, I don't mind, you know, but it's the silly ones, the ones that say it's a pity they can't do something when they're small, you know—when they're born. Well, I think that's ridiculous, because she's a happy child—and they more or less think that they shouldn't let them live—well, I think that's wrong.

Boy: 4 yrs.

Only the sort of advice you get from people who are nosy—*that* sort of advice . . . I doubt whether anybody would *not* get advice like that—I'm always getting it! I've had advice like, 'Tie his right arm back so that he's got to use his left arm', which would be cruel, extremely cruel. Then, of course, you get the nasty sort of people who say that children like that ought to be done away with.

Girl: 7 yrs.

I wouldn't like it if they didn't. I don't want her to be ignored just because she isn't normal.

Boy: 6 yrs.

Well, I think you've *got* to talk about the child. I mean, they're there and that's all there is to it. You can't hide these children. That's the wrong attitude.

Boy: 6 yrs.

Oh, I don't dislike it, no. In fact, I suppose I'm a bit peculiar, but it doesn't bother me that I've got a handicapped child. I think if people are going to be funny about it, I just don't want to know them, because I think it's such a silly attitude.

Boy: 6 yrs.

I don't think it's right that every time you stop, the children should sit and hear themselves being talked about.

Boy: 2½ yrs. (Pilot study)

It doesn't bother me. It embarrasses them more than it does me.

The point made by the last speaker is an important one. Many mothers sense that people who have normal children only, feel embarrassed and afraid of hurting their feelings and so avoid contact. As we have seen, so long as the interest shown is not merely morbid curiosity, it is more likely to be welcomed than not. For some mothers, of course, equanimity in the face of friends and of curious strangers has been hardly won over a period of time. The comments of two of the mothers seen at the pilot stage of the project may be of interest to new mothers who have not yet achieved it.

Girl: 2 yrs. (Pilot study)

I've sort of hibernated, really, since I've known about her, I'm coming out a little bit more now because, of course, I think time heals, you know, just a little bit; but, I mean, when she was having these awful convulsions, I couldn't take her out then. I'd no sooner get down the road and she'd start going into one of these awful convulsions—I was *terrified* I was going to meet someone I knew. In fact, I've been at the top of the road and seen somebody p'raps talking to somebody else down there and I've waited around till I've seen them gone and then come. My husband gets cross with me because he says anybody would think she's some monstrosity, but it's seeing the other babies, you know. They've probably got their children and that hurts a lot. I never thought I'd have to go through it.

Girl: 6 yrs. (Pilot study)

I like them to talk about her. I must admit that when she was about a year old I felt a bit 'difficult'—but once everybody knew, I found it a lot easier. Once they *knew* that she wasn't normal, I found it a lot easier to talk about it then.

Most mothers find the people who stare at their children unacceptable, although some have a robust approach even to this:

Boy: 7 yrs.

Well, I just don't care what other people think about it. When I take him a walk, when they're standing staring and that, it doesn't bother me. I know he's my lad and I love him. I don't care about anybody else.

The replies of the East Midlands mothers to these questions seem to indicate that, given a sensible and understanding public who take an intelligent interest, mothers of handicapped children would be more than willing to meet such interest half way —they will do their part if we will. They are only too anxious to have their children accepted as members of the community.

Some have found that even their near relatives are non-plussed by the difficulties of handling handicapped children and so lack the confidence to offer to care for them for short periods. In spite of this, however, parents of the handicapped children seemed to go out together as often as parents of the normal 4-year-olds, according to their replies to questions about use of baby-sitters. The questions asked were the same for both samples and Table 5.III shows their responses. In addition, the responses

TABLE 5.III

Frequency of use of baby-sitters

	Normal 1-yr.-olds N = 700	Normal 4-yr.-olds N = 700	E. Midlands C.P.s N = 180
1 p.w. or more	22%	25%	18%
1 per month ⎱ Seldom ⎰	38%	16% ⎱ 26% ⎰ 42%	19% ⎱ 23% ⎰ 42%
1 p.a. or never	40%	33%	40%
	100%	100%	100%

TABLE 5.IV

Who baby-sits?

	Normal 4-yr.-olds	E. Midlands C.P.s
Paid sitter	16%	12%
Unpaid sitter	59%	61%
Older sibs	19%	25%
Inadequate arrangements	6%	2%
	100%	100%

of the normal children's parents who were interviewed at the 1-year-old stage have been included—these are of interest as some of the East Midlands children were under 4 years old, and some were needing to be cared for as though they were much younger than their actual age.

There is no evidence here to suggest that the presence of a handicapped child radically alters normal patterns of joint outings for the parents. It is true that some mothers said that they felt that it was difficult to find anyone really capable of caring for their children, particularly if the child was subject to fits (these are very alarming for anyone who is not accustomed to them), but their attitudes in general were very similar to those of parents of normal 1-year-old children. These parents, too, often expressed doubts about the competence of baby-sitters and there were other similarities between them and the parents of the handicapped children that are worth looking at.[1]

1. *Normal 1-year-olds:* Oh, no, we never go out—my husband would never go out—he wouldn't let anyone come in and let us both go out.
   E. Midlands C.P.s.: Never, my husband don't believe in it. He was left so much as a child himself.
2. *Normal 1-year-olds:* Not unless I know them properly. I've got to know the person and trust them.
   E. Midlands C.P.s: No. My husband won't leave her, only with my mother. He feels she's the only one capable.
3. *Normal 1-year-olds:* We don't believe in it. We think if you have children you should take that responsibility and look after them yourself all the time.
   E. Midlands C.P.s: Before I had any I always said—you know, you get people leaving them with people, going out, but it never worries me. I've always said that they're my responsibility and that's it.
4. *Normal 1-year olds:* We never do—much to my disgust. The children won't put up with it, I'm afraid—they just cry. And then, between the two of them, I've never felt it's fair to burden anyone with them if they're going to cry all night.
   E. Midlands C.P.s: He seems to know if I'm going out and he cries the place down, so I never go now.

The last comment shows that it is not only mothers of the handicapped who defer to their children's wishes in this respect. On the other hand, some parents of handicapped children are so aware of the possibility that their children could become very dependent on them that they are willing to go out in spite of the child's objections:

Boy: 7 yrs.

At one time, when we went out at night, if we had a sitter in, we used to have an awful job with him. He used to scream and didn't want us to go. He'd sort of relied on us so much. But we sort of persevered with going out. We thought, 'Well, we can't go on with him clinging to one person like this.' And then when he got about

---

[1] Similar comments are not available for the 4-year-old sample.

five he'd say, 'When are you going to go out, Mummy, so that Granny can come and look after us?'

Girl: 6 yrs.

She still cries a bit but I just have to leave her, 'cos they always say, 'Don't turn back then 'cos she knows—when you get up the street she stops, but if you turn back she goes bad again.' They always tell me to go, 'cos I used to turn back and wouldn't go and it made me that I never got out.

Fourteen of the East Midlands mothers said that baby-sitting was one kind of help they would have liked that they hadn't had, and six of these specified *trained* baby-sitters with special understanding of the needs of handicapped children. In the words of one of them:

You see, the point is not just having *someone* to take the child for an hour or two hours, but having someone that you know can cope. Someone who understands spastics and won't let them fall and bang their heads or something dangerous. Because your whole fear is, when they're small, with someone like Alastair, that they'll damage their right hand (i.e. the 'good' one) or something like that, and then what would you do for him? Well, having anyone else to take them out or to their house and that, you don't worry *all* the time but you don't feel as happy as if you knew they were with someone who knew about spastics.

However, this reaction is a minority one, and if parents do not go out it is more likely to be because they have the same attitudes as any other parents than because it is made more difficult for them. A definite social class trend was revealed in attitudes to leaving the children with baby-sitters in the study of normal children at the 1-year-old stage. Working class fathers, in particular, were reported by their wives to 'lay down the law' in this respect, and insist that the children should not be left except possibly with one of their grandparents. 'You don't have kiddies to leave 'em.' 'Our turn will come when they're grown up.' These were two of the comments quoted to illustrate this very general attitude.[1] There were instances of the same general attitudes operating in the East Midlands sample, sometimes to the exasperation of the mother, as in the following comment (the same mother is speaking as in the first comparison of attitudes above):

[1] Newson, J. & E., op. cit., 1963.

I should love a night out, you know. I mean, my husband—he doesn't understand my side at all. He's at work all day and has a laugh and a joke with the men and that. He's quite happy to come home and sit in, you know. But I'm here all the time. I should love a night out. I mean, always he's said, 'We can't leave the children.' We'd never leave them on their own—I wouldn't. But now . . . (the eldest boy) is going into 15 we could easy put the others to bed and him sit and listen, like, and watch the telly. But me husband won't. He's a proper stay-at-home. *I* am—*I'm* a stay-at-home. I enjoy me home—but you can have *too* much.

But baby-sitting problems do not necessarily mean that parents do not go out at all, since 59% of mothers said that they went out without their husbands, and a similar number that their husbands went out alone. This might only mean a drink at the 'local' for fathers, or a weekly visit to 'me Mam' for the mothers, although many had a much wider range of interests and activities, often pursued independently of husband or wife.

Baby-sitting, as discussed above, has meant having someone to care for the child in his own home, usually after he has gone to bed. Leaving children to be cared for in other people's homes, particularly during the day, probably *is* more difficult for parents of handicapped children. Comparison with figures for the normal 4-year-olds shows that whereas 11% of the normal children were left elsewhere[1] as often as twice or more per week, only 6% of the East Midlands children were left this often. This difference, although not very great, is significant statistically[2] and may be an indication of the lack of confidence in their ability to handle the handicapped child, which is felt by some grandparents and other relatives or neighbours. Comments by some of the mothers who had met this difficulty show that their efforts to lead a normal life are sometimes hampered by the attitudes of their relations.

Boy: 8 yrs.

My mother-in-law, it upsets her. She doesn't like to see him. She says it upsets her to see him. She went on holiday with us this year and I think we left him with her about 10 minutes and took the other children to a little playground—oh, she couldn't manage him, you know, she said he was crying and she said 'Oh, I couldn't

---

[1] This does not include attendance at nursery schools and play-groups.
[2] $\chi^2 = 3.93$, $\eta = 1$, $P < .05$.

manage him.' He's a big boy now, a good 8-year-old—*my* mother's had him quite a bit but he's getting too much for *her*, now. He's been to stop odd times, but she's not very big and he gets a bit strong now.

Boy: 6 yrs.

I've never had any help from my family or my husband's family. As for my friends, I have only one who goes out of her way to take an interest in him. She's the only one I would really trust him with in my absence . . . (Interviewer: You wouldn't leave him with your relations?) No, because I don't think they could cope, you know, because they're more for institutionalizing such as him— you know, not very sympathetic—more sympathetic to me than to him. They think that I'm depriving myself and all that business.

Boy: 4 yrs.

Actually, my mother and I had a terrific row, you see. She told me I should let him go away, you see, permanently, and I said I wasn't going to. She didn't speak to me for six months.

Turning now from the consideration of opportunities for parents to go out without their children, what can be said about those occasions when parents and children usually go out together? The family holiday, for example, although it is historically a recent phenomenon for the majority of the working population, is already very much taken for granted in many families. Perhaps the presence of a handicapped child seriously interferes with this activity. Special schemes are in operation which are based on this premise and which offer various ways of overcoming the difficulties. We asked the East Midlands mothers what their experience regarding holidays had been since the birth of the handicapped child. One hundred and twenty-eight of them (71%) had been on holiday at least once, taking their handicapped child with them. Of these, the majority (64% of the whole sample) had found their holiday accommodation in the usual ways, many of them staying in caravans at coastal resorts—an increasingly popular solution to the problems of expense for all families, not only those with handicapped children. But all the other possibilities were reported as well—hotels, boarding houses, bungalows, holiday camps, staying with relations and friends who lived near the coast or in other desirable locations. The remaining 13 families (7% of the whole sample) had spent their holidays in special accommodation provided by various bodies (such as local groups of the Spastics Society)—caravans, holiday flats or bungalows.

The fact that so many families had managed to take their handicapped children away with them did not mean that all such holidays were an unqualified success, of course, and there was a considerable number of mothers who would have been glad of an opportunity to take a holiday without the handicapped child. We asked whether the children had been offered special holidays for handicapped children, without their parents. We also asked whether they had accepted such holidays and whether they *would* accept if they were offered in the future. The replies in Table 5.V refer specifically to real holidays and do not include offers of short-term care in Family Help Units or other institutions.

TABLE 5.V

Use and potential use of special holiday schemes

Special holiday for handicapped children	*No. of children*	
Child had been	12 ⎫	
Offered; but mother refused outright	12 ⎬ 21%	
Offered; mother would accept later	13 ⎭	
Not offered; mother would accept now	38 ⎫ 44%	
Not offered; mother would accept when child is older	42 ⎭	
Not offered; mother undecided, or would not accept	63	35%
	180	100%

Less than a quarter of the mothers said that they had been offered holidays for their children, whereas rather more than half said that they would accept such a holiday some time if it should be offered, probably when the children were old enough not to mind being away from home and to enjoy the company of other children. Most of those who were not interested in such help had only slightly handicapped children, or children who seemed to be so little aware of, or affected by, their surroundings that there seemed to be no point in it. Some felt that their children would not enjoy being away from their families.

There were 25 families (14% of the whole sample) who simply could not afford to take a holiday away from their own homes, and some of these mothers said that they had never had a holiday since they had been married, or even in their whole lives. The fact that one of their children was handicapped made no difference whatsoever to the situation. Provision of temporary care or of a special holiday with the handicapped child would not necessarily help such mothers—the care of the other children would still be a difficulty, even if the mother could accept the idea of being away from her family, an idea so foreign to many of them that they would have to be desperate indeed to entertain it.

Only 4 of the remaining families who had not taken a holiday together said that they had been prevented from doing so because of the difficulty of finding suitable accommodation. In 11 instances, other circumstances had kept the family at home, moving house, for example, or the birth of another baby.

We have no comparable data about family holidays from the study of normal 4-year-olds.

It is sometimes suggested in the literature that handicapped children are taken out less frequently than are normal children. For this reason, the East Midlands mothers were also asked questions about the kinds of outings on which they took their children, apart from shopping and visiting relations. There is again no comparable data available from the study of normal 4-year-olds (but the 7-year-old stage of that study will yield information on this point). The experience of all children in this respect, handicapped and normal alike, must be affected by a number of circumstances such as the area in which they live and the amenities offered there, the number of children in the family and whether there is a car available to solve transport problems[1] and, above all, the preferences, tastes and finances of the particular family. The answers to these questions, therefore, tended to vary widely. For the purpose of analysis, they were grouped into 5 categories, 3 of which are self-explanatory. Those considered to indicate a 'wide' or a 'narrow' range of outings are best illustrated by examples of the variety of outings which would justify inclusion in either category, in particular cases.

1. Examples of 'wide' range of outings:

Girl, 3 yrs.: 2 younger children, living in rural area near coast: visiting friends, local places of interest, e.g. Thornton Abbey, to the beach, 'everywhere, we go all over'—family has a car.

[1] 53% of the sample owned cars. This compares with about 50% of all private households in the East Midlands (Census (10%) 1966) which was in its turn above the national average of about 40%.

Boy, 8 *yrs.*: no other children, living in rural area near coast: swimming, caravanning, cinema, cricket, motor-scrambling—family has a car.

Boy, 6 *yrs.*: 6 older children, living in inland rural area: taken for walks, to nearby city, mother's son-in-law takes for rides in his car to find trains to watch, takes to zoo in next county—family has no car.

2. Examples of 'narrow' range of outings:

Boy, 3 *yrs.*: 2 younger children, living near small market town: visiting relatives, occasionally to coast—family has a car.

Girl, 3 *yrs.*: 1 brother several years older, living in a city area: taken occasionally to visit relatives, to beauty spots in neighbouring county—family has a car.

Boy, 5 *yrs.*: 4 younger children, living in a city area; taken to local park, for walks, to see friends—family has no car.

These examples show that the terms 'narrow' and 'wide' refer more to the variety of experiences made available to the child than to actual distances travelled. Table 5.VI shows the distri-

TABLE 5.VI

Range of outings and car ownership

	Family has car	No car	Total percentage
	Number of children		
Unaffected by handicap[1]	10	9	11%
Wide range	44	14	32%
Narrow range	37	37	41%
Walking distance only	1	19	11%
Seldom goes out	3	6	5%
	95	85	100%

[1] Includes all ranges of outings, but handicap is obviously not a factor in these instances.

bution of replies to these questions and also whether the family owned a car. As can be seen from these figures, owning a car does not automatically mean that the family has a wide variety of outings. However, when the figures are broken down according to degree of physical and mental handicap (Table 5.VII), a pattern emerges that suggests that parental behaviour in respect of taking children out is modified more by the presence or absence of a car than by severity of handicap. For example, in

TABLE 5.VII

Range of outings

Related to car ownership and degree of handicap

Degree of handicap	CAR					NO CAR					Total
	Seldom goes out	Walking distance only	Narrow range	Wide range	Unaffected by handicap	Seldom goes out	Walking distance only	Narrow range	Wide range	Unaffected by handicap	
Minimal to mild	0	0 ⎱0	7	22 ⎱29	8	1	3 ⎱4	20	8 ⎱28	8	77
Moderate	0	1 ⎱1	10	10 ⎱20	1	2	8 ⎱10	7	2 ⎱9	0	41
Severe	3	0 ⎱3	20	12 ⎱32	1	3	8 ⎱11	10	4 ⎱14	1	62
											180
Mental status											
'Normal'	0	0 ⎱0	7	10 ⎱17	6	1	0 ⎱1	10	4 ⎱14	7	45
Uncertain	1	0 ⎱1	10	16 ⎱26	3	3	7 ⎱10	10	7 ⎱17	1	58
Confirmed defect	2	1 ⎱3	15	15 ⎱30	1	1	11 ⎱12	16	1 ⎱17	0	63
Main handicap mental	0	0 ⎱0	5	3 ⎱8	0	1	1 ⎱2	1	2 ⎱3	1	14
											180

the group with 'minimal to mild' physical handicap ratings, ownership of a car reverses the pattern of the range of outings but does not significantly affect the overall numbers, whereas in the group with 'severe' physical handicap ratings, the pattern is only very slightly altered but the numbers taken on a more than very limited range of outings are twice as large in the car-owning group. Even the very slightly handicapped are much more restricted in their outings if the family has no car.

Finally, we have to consider the question of opportunity to meet and interact with children other than their own brothers and sisters. Here we do have a little information about the normal 4-year-olds which will serve as a basis for comparison. The East Midlands mothers were asked whether the other children in the family brought home friends to play, and if so, whether the handicapped child was included at all in their play and/or conversation. They were also asked whether the other children ever took them out to play in the street or park, and whether they ever went to play in other children's houses. On the basis of replies to these questions and on the number of days per week each child attended school or day-centre, they were judged to have wide contacts with other children (43%), restricted contacts (38%) or minimal contacts (19%). Of the 19% considered to have only minimal contacts, 9 were attending day-centre for one or two days per week. Thus, discounting these 9 children, 13% of the East Midlands handicapped children were very restricted in their contacts with other children while only 7% of the normal Nottingham 4-year-olds were so restricted; the normal families also had the prospect of school, which would eliminate this problem in the near future. Some of the handicapped children were already well past school age but no suitable day care had been arranged for them. Their experiences at home seemed to be very limited. This means that a small proportion of the East Midlands sample were seriously deprived of opportunities for social learning, 9 children of 5 years or more and 14 who were under 5 years. Numerically the problem may seem to be insignificant. This does not lessen its impact for the individuals concerned.

There was evidence that the home life of some of the children who were considered to have only minimal contacts with children other than their own brothers and sisters, was curtailed in other ways as well. Seventeen of them spent much of the day

in special chairs, in prams, or similarly confined in a safe place
of some kind. Of this 17, 11 spent much of their time in one room,
the living room of their homes. These 11 children were, with one
exception, severely handicapped physically and/or mentally—
the exceptional child had moderate physical handicaps. Their
ages ranged from 2 years to 7 years. If parents of such children
seem to be at a loss to know how to introduce variety into their
lives, an example of the experience of one of them may go some
way to explain why this is so. This mother described her 7-year-
old daughter as 'just like a 7-month-old baby' (and this seemed
to the interviewer to be a fair comment). In addition to her
other handicaps, this little girl was blind. Her only pleasure was
to listen to music and rock back and forth in her chair. She was
a poor sleeper and a problem to feed, taking liquid foods only.
She was taken for walks but not on other outings—the family
had no car. Her parents rarely went out together because she
woke up screaming 3 or 4 times most nights, but they did go
out separately, mother to 'Bingo' and father to the 'local' for a
drink. Her mother was one of those who felt lonely and had no
friends, but she had some contact with her mother and sister.
She also said she often felt depressed. In spite of all these circumstances, this mother said that she was not anxious for her
daughter to have day-care because she was not convinced that
the care available would be any better than, or even as good as,
her own. The child had only been away from home once, when
she was 5 years old, for 3 weeks of temporary care while the
mother was not well. During these 3 weeks, she had been cared
for mainly in a cot in a quiet room, so that it had taken 3 weeks
after going back home for her to get used to ordinary household
noises again. There seemed no doubt that however restricted
the child's life was at home, she was more in contact with people
and with ordinary life there than she would have been in any
but the most specialized institutional setting.

Interaction with other children can involve not only playing
together but also quarrelling. Information is available as to the
extent that mothers are prepared to encourage their normal
4-year-olds to settle their own differences and 'stick up for
themselves', if necessary by using force. Where appropriate,
similar information was obtained for the East Midlands children but only 60% of the sample could be included, the question
being irrelevant to the remaining 40% because they were too

young, too handicapped or too isolated to become involved in quarrels. However, the tendency to encourage their children to hit back is shown for both samples in Table 5.VIII.

TABLE 5.VIII

Mothers' encouragement to 'hit back'

	Normal 4-year-olds N = 700	East Midlands Sample N = 109
Never	18%	16%
Yes, qualified	21% } 82%	12% } 84%
Yes, unambiguous	61%	72%

Once more the two groups gave very similar responses. The majority of the East Midlands mothers, where the question was relevant, considered that their children were behaving quite adequately in this respect. Eleven of them thought their children were too passive in their approach to quarrels, and 15 that their children tended to be aggressive. However, 11 of the mothers of aggressive children still found it necessary to encourage them to defend themselves.

Basic attitudes to leaving the children to sort out their own quarrels and arguments were apparent in both groups of mothers when discussing the problem of quarrels with children outside the family. Parents commented over and over again that 'you can't fall out over your kids', if only because while the parents are occupied with trying to sort out the rights and wrongs of their children's disputes, perhaps with some acrimony between neighbours, the children are busy 'making it up' again. There were mothers in both samples who also pointed out, that although they would have preferred not to encourage retaliation, they were forced into it by the behaviour of the neighbouring children.

The two groups of handicapped children who seemed to have the most difficulty fitting into the ordinary play situation with normal children, were those whose physical handicaps were just severe enough to make it impossible to keep up with the others in all their activities, but not severe enough for the other children to make allowances for them, and the mentally handicapped who, although mobile enough to play, lacked the understanding necessary for acceptable social interaction. Some examples of these difficulties follow:

Boy: 8 yrs.

Sometimes he'll find that he'll go out, thrilled to bits because we've let him go and then about 10 minutes later he comes back and he's real down in the mouth; he'll say, 'They wouldn't stop with me.' We've talked to him about it, we've told him it's understandable—boys especially; girls will play with him more, naturally. With the boys, we find that they'll play with him half an hour, then he can't race about, so gradually he's left on his own and he comes home—'It's not fair, nobody will play with me'.

Boy: 5 yrs. (mentally handicapped)

He doesn't mix with normal children at all, he just pulls their hair and pushes them, you see, and you can't ask them to your home with children. He's very friendly but he will pull hair, that's his trouble and children are frightened of him . . . he pulls his daddy's hair terrible and he's had some smacks! . . . He loves other children—he puts his arms towards them to love them and then changes his mind and pulls—he's not nasty with it—I don't really know what he does feel about it . . . I think they do need other children's company—he comes home from the Mount (The Family Help Unit) on Tuesday absolutely tired out and happy as can be and you can tell that he's been playing with the other children. He gets frustrated here all the time—I can't play with him all the time.

The child who is more handicapped physically may not always have these problems. The mother of one such boy, who at 5+ was attending an ordinary school, said, 'Of course, all the kiddies make a fuss of him. They all run to push him in and push him out and give him his milk, you know, and things like that. They're all very good.' This mother seemed to be very happy about her son's acceptance at school. He was one of a large family and had older brothers and sisters who took an interest in him as well. Although he was not yet able to walk, he was certainly not deprived of the companionship of other children. However, the problem of company for the children is not an easy one for mothers to solve if the family is small and the child is not going daily to school or day-centre. Other children cannot be coerced into playing with one who cannot take his full part in games, even though the mother may be well aware that he needs their company. 'He loves parties and laughter and people—joins in and really enjoys himself. He loves people around him—the more the better. I think it's because he's so bored on his own that he likes attention and lots of laughter and gaiety.' The mother speaking here has a physically and mentally handicapped boy who, at almost 7 years old, was not going daily to a day-centre, but who was 'really happy' on the two days per week that he went to the Family Help Unit. At home he had only one infant sister and no opportunities to see other children, but the problem of providing the companionship he needed could not be solved by his mother's own efforts. If such a child were later deemed to be 'socially immature', it would hardly be fair to lay the entire responsibility for this on his family or his handicap. There is ample evidence provided by the East Midlands mothers, that they are in the main well aware of their children's needs, but that some of them need more help from community services to enable them, and the family as a whole, to lead the normal life they strive to achieve.

CHAPTER 6

EDUCATION, TRAINING AND DAY-CARE

Unlike ordinary children, they cannot acquire, in the course of their daily explorations and activities, all the essential information they need in order to be ready to benefit from schooling at the age of 5 years. They must be given preliminary training in the pre-school years and special education at school.

MARY SHERIDAN[1]

Perhaps the handicapped child is deprived most of all of early contact with his peers.

ROBERT WIGGLESWORTH[2]

The provision of suitable education, training or day-care is generally acknowledged to be of paramount importance for the handicapped child. Statements like those above occur over and over again in the literature about handicapped children of all kinds and that which deals with cerebral palsy is no exception. There is usually special emphasis on the advantages to the child and to his family that can accrue when education or training starts before the child is of normal school age, particularly when his handicaps are of a kind that seriously restrict his everyday experiences. The fact that for some children it is not only desirable but essential to begin their education well before the usual age of 5 years was acknowledged when the 1944 Education Act included the provision that, whenever it seems likely that a child will need special educational provision, both the local authority and the parents themselves have the right to request

---

[1] Op. cit.
[2] Wigglesworth, Robert. 'The Value of Early Part-time Developmental Training' in *The Spastic School Child and the Outside World*. Eds. James Loring and Anita Mason. The Spastics Society—Heinemann, London, 1966.

that he is presented for formal ascertainment of his needs at any time after he is 2 years old. The person most likely to suggest that this is necessary is the hospital consultant or the family doctor. It is very unusual for parents to be aware that they have this right.

In order to 'ascertain' a child's special educational needs, or indeed to establish the existence of such needs in particular instances, 'careful preliminary observation, with full medical examination and psychological assessment, carried out by specially experienced medical officers and educational psychologists, who are authorized by the Department of Education and Science for the purpose'[1] is necessary. In practice, when this happens at all, it happens most often when the child's fifth birthday is imminent. The decision will then be taken either to include the child in the ordinary school system, to offer special education for him in a special school or class, or, if he is deemed to be 'unsuitable for education at a school' (what used to be called 'ineducable') to exclude him from the school system altogether. If he is so excluded, responsibility for his training falls to the health authority, not the education authority, although there is reason to believe that this is to be changed in the foreseeable future,[2] and discussions are proceeding at ministerial level which should make the education of all children the responsibility of local education authorities. At the time of interview parents had the right to appeal to the Minister of Education within 21 days of being notified of such a decision to exclude a child, if they wish to dispute it for any reason. They were also entitled to have the child re-assessed at 12-monthly intervals and to make a further appeal on each occasion, if necessary.

Seventy-eight children in the sample (43%) had been examined or 'ascertained' by local authorities, 52 of them by someone who was thought by the mother to have been a psychologist, and 26 by school medical officers.[3] (The doubt as to the status of the person administering the tests arises as part of the general uncertainty parents experience about the identity of the different workers with whom they are brought into contact.) Nine of these children had also been assessed by the

---

[1] Dr Mary Sheridan in *The Handicapped Child and his Home* (op. cit.).
[2] At the time of writing—September 1968.
[3] All of these children were older than three years when they were ascertained— i.e. they were not ascertained before nursery school age.

Spastics Society in London, and one by the Spastics Centre at Cheyne Walk, Chelsea.

The Spastics Society had assessed 22 of the children in all, including the 9 cited above. Cheyne Walk Centre had seen 3 children in all, and Great Ormond Street Hospital, a Rudolf Steiner home, a local authority 'mental health clinic' (so described by the mother) and a private specialist had each seen one child.

The major role, then, in the testing of handicapped children is played by the local authorities, and parents seem to be aware that the procedures used are intended more to discover which children shall be excluded from the school system than to attempt to assess the extent of a child's capabilities, however limited, and to provide suitable education for him. The decision is often made after a brief visit to the child at home, or an interview at a clinic, and bears little resemblance to the 'long period of observation by a team of experts' which Dr Mary Sheridan (op. cit.) and others suggest is often necessary.

The problem is not always solved from the parents' point of view by taking the child to London for assessment by a voluntary body. They feel that a long journey, and possibly an overnight stay in strange surroundings, are not the best kind of preliminary to an assessment which may have very far-reaching implications for both parents and children.

Re assessments away from home

Boy: 8 yrs.

> At the Spastics Society in London, he was frightened to death. He wouldn't do anything at all . . . so we waited and took him again and they said although he'd improved, he hadn't improved enough to warrant them placing him anywhere. In other words, progress was going to be very, very slow and they hadn't got time for him. They only seem to want the ones they say would make a success afterwards.

Girl: 5 yrs.

> She wouldn't do anything for them. My husband said it was a waste of time going—she wouldn't say a word to them! They said she could go this year some time—they suggested travelling by night, but you're still going to be as bad off, aren't you?

Girl: 7 yrs.

It's a terrible feeling when you *know* she can do it, it really is . . .
Next time we go to London, if they reject her, I shall have something to say, because I think she should at least have the chance of
an assessment centre where she can stay for a couple of days,
because honestly, there's many a normal child—you take them to
new surroundings, strange surroundings, and they won't do a
quarter of what they can do at home.

Re local authority ascertainment

Girl: 7 yrs.

I'm afraid we're not awfully thrilled with the way they go about the
assessment. Of course, all they're testing for is a normal school, I
suppose. They're assessing them for what they've got available in
the country, aren't they? . . . We find the assessment is wholly a
farce, really, the way it's done, because obviously she can't do a
normal assessment because of her inability to use her hands and
things. They should really have special sorts of assessment for
children like this. All it tells them is, they're not fit for a normal
school, it doesn't tell them how much there is there, you know, for
a special school.

Boy: 7 yrs.

Well, they just said they haven't passed him at all, and a few weeks
ago I wrote to the M.O.H. and asked them if she'd test him. I got
a letter back to say that she would and then the mental welfare
officer came and she said it was a waste of time. I thought it was
a test to see if he could go to a special school, but apparently it
isn't, it's only to see if—they thought I wanted him to go to a
normal school—so anyway, they said don't bother with the test,
it'll not do any good. He'll not go to a normal school.

Girl: 7 yrs.

I had a letter saying the child psychologist was coming to see her.
Well, when she came she said 'I don't know what they've sent me
to see her for.' She could see she couldn't possibly go to school,
not even the centre, you know. She was very indignant . . . She
was cn the floor, like this, and they just asked me a few questions.
She said, 'She needs institutional care.' That's what she said.

The real problems arise, not for parents whose children are
ascertained as educable and for whom educational provision is
made, nor for those who are so obviously and severely handi-

capped that even their parents find it difficult to elicit responses of any kind, but for those parents who find their children more responsive in their own environment than they are in test situations. Perhaps such children would respond well if they were assessed at home over a period of time by someone with special skill and competence. The problem then would be to provide suitable placement for them.

With regard to the comments quoted above, two things should be emphasized. The first is obvious—we do not know the views of parents whose children have been 'successful' in the assessment situation and who have gone to boarding school as a result. We only have the views of those who have been less fortunate. Parents who are satisfied and whose children go to special schools have far less to say on the subject, although one mother whose child had been assessed at school said 'They were pretty thorough. They were there all morning.' It is the rule rather than the exception for parents of *any* child to be dissatisfied with intelligence testing procedures. The 'standardized situation' represents a hurdle for all children, but this is even more true for the handicapped, for many reasons. They are therefore more likely to do themselves less than justice in the test situation than are normal children.

Secondly, in response to the kind of criticism we have quoted, the Spastics Society have recently opened an assessment centre in London where families can stay, so giving child and parents a chance to settle down and relax.

When a child has been 'ascertained' as being in need of special educational provision, the local authority has an obligation to make such provision. In practice, however, there are not enough special school places, and far from starting their education earlier than normal children, those who are mentally and/ or physically handicapped often have to wait until they are well over 5 years old before a suitable place is provided for them. The overall number of children in England and Wales ascertained as being in need of special educational provision has been rising: in 1963 the total number of such children, both in schools and waiting for places was 88,036; in 1965 it was 95,528. The size of the waiting list does not vary very much; 13,108 were waiting for places in 1963, 13,169 in 1965. In both instances, about 95 % of these children were 5 years old or older. The number of children who have been waiting for more than a year is going down a little, having been reduced by about 1,000 since 1963, when it was 6,030.[1] All these figures refer to children who have been ascertained as in need of special educational treatment, and do not include those who have been excluded from the school system altogether.

In the area called the North Midlands by the Department of Education and Science, which corresponds to the area that we have called the East Midlands, 4,445 pupils, or 0.7% of school-age children, were being catered for in 61 special schools in 1965. The number so catered for over England and Wales as a whole was 1% of the total number of school-age children.[2]

It is well known that education authorities have the right to prosecute parents who fail to send their children to school when they reach the age of 5, or who fail to convince the authority that they have provided suitable alternative education. The converse, however, does not seem to be the case, and authorities who continue to fail to fulfill their statutory obligations to handicapped children appear to do so with impunity.

Given this national situation with regard to special education, it is not surprising that for many parents of handicapped children, the difficulty of obtaining suitable education or day-care for them is a primary source of anxiety. Table 6.I shows the range of education and day-care which had been provided for the East Midlands sample at the time of interview. When considering the figures in this table, it must be remembered that it does not take into account any kind of residential provision that has been made for children of this age group in the East Midlands area. These are all children who were being cared for at home, with one exception—in the 'other' column there is one child who had just started his first term at boarding school when his mother was interviewed. It was decided to retain this child in the sample as he had actually been away from his home for a shorter period than had some of the children who were in temporary care at the time of interview.

There were 125 children in the sample who were 5 years old or older at the time of interview. Twenty six of them were having no education or day care of any kind. Another 19 were attending for one or two days per week at centres provided by voluntary bodies (notably the Spastics Society in Nottingham and else-

---

[1] Statistics of Education, H.M.S.O., 1965 and 1966.
[2] Statistics of Education, H.M.S.O., 1965 and 1966.

Table 6.I

Educational provision and day-care

Mental Status of Children	None	Ord. school	Special school	5-day boarder	1–2 days p.w. at centre	3+ days p.w. at centre	Home teacher < 5 hrs. p.w.	Home teacher 5 hrs. + p.w.	Other	Total
					Number of Children					
Normal										
Aged 5+	1	26	4	1	—	—	2	1	1	36
Under 5	5	—	—	—	3	—	—	—	—	9
Uncertain										
Aged 5+	4	2	6	1	3	4	2	—	1	23
Under 5	22	1	—	—	10	2	—	—	—	35
Confirmed mental handicap										
Aged 5+	21	3	3	2	16	18	—	1	4	68*
Under 5	7	—	—	—	2	1	—	—	1	11
Total	60	32	13	4	34*	25	4	2	8	N=180

* Two children appear twice here. One goes to a day-centre 2 days per week and also has a home teacher for 5 hours per week. The other goes to a day-centre 1 day per week and also has 2 home teachers for 5 hours each per week.

where but there were others) and one went to a private nursery school. This means that 37% of the school age children were not provided for in any way by the local authorities concerned. According to their mothers' reports, 4 only of these children were on waiting lists for residential provision.

Of the 55 children who were under 5 years old, 34 or 62% were having no nursery day-care of any kind. Sixteen were going for 1 or 2 days per week to centres run by voluntary bodies (again largely the Spastics Society). This leaves 5 'under-fives' who were being provided with pre-school training or care by local authorities (10% of the 2–4 year olds).

The mothers in the East Midlands Sample appeared to be well aware that handicapped children are as much in need of the company of companions their own age, and of the stimulus of an environment other than their own homes as are normal children. Most of them clearly recognize that children can become too dependent on them unless they are given opportunities to learn independence. They also realize that they themselves can become too involved with their children. This problem of inter-dependence between mother and child—and it is important to remember that it *is* a two-way process, for mothers of normal as well as of handicapped children—is solved automatically for mothers and their normal children when school time comes at 5, but although the enforced break is welcome in a general sort of way, many mothers miss their children when they first start school. (Indeed, one mother in the East Midlands sample explained that she had planned her family of three children so that there was always a baby arriving in time to fill the gap left by the 5-year-old starting school.) For many mothers of handicapped children, an already intensified situation of inter-dependence is prolonged. A mother caring for a 6-year-old who still behaves like a young baby in most respects, has no alternative but to go on mothering him as though he really were a baby, even though she can see the perils of this situation both for herself and the child, particularly when no day-care is offered.

Most of the mothers of these children, including the nursery age children, said that they would like to have some sort of day-care for them. There is evidence that there is a large unfulfilled demand for nursery schools for all children, so that the mothers of the handicapped children are by no means unusual in this respect.[1] (As far as the normal children are concerned, there has been a government embargo on the expansion of nursery schools and classes until deficiencies in schooling for 5+ children have been rectified, which has only been lifted to accommodate the children of married women teachers returning to the profession; but this does not apply to those children who until now have been outside the normal educational system, and whose needs should be catered for under the National Health Service Act, once they have been 'ascertained' under the Education Act.) This does not mean, however, that mothers will accept without protest or criticism the present standards of provision for severely handicapped children even when it is offered. Some of them are well aware that 'the contrast between the type of education given to mentally handicapped children and to normal children of about the same level of development is a very striking one.'[2] Some expressed the view that children were given more attention at home than at under-staffed day-centres. Others thought that the sight of children more severely handicapped than they were themselves was disturbing for their children, and that they were inclined to imitate the bizarre gestures and sounds made by such children. Some mothers commented that junior training centres were misnamed because the children were *not* trained or taught at all, but went merely in order to give their mothers a rest, and expressed their feeling that local authorities are not sufficiently interested in those who are excluded from the school system, a belief which is reinforced[3] when a long time is allowed to elapse between the child's fifth birthday and his admission to a training centre or special care unit. Some of their comments on this topic follow:

Boy: 5 yrs.

I would like him to go to a training centre; when they're 5 they definitely should go somewhere because they need the company of other children and it's only right that there should be somewhere for them to go. Normal children go away when they're 5, to school. And *we* need a break—I think we need a break more than the

[1] See E. Newson. 'Provision for the Pre-School Child' in *Graduate Women at Work*. Ed. Constance E. Arregger.

[2] Tizard, J. *Community Services for the Mentally Handicapped*. O.U.P., London, 1964.

[3] Professor Tizard comments, too, on the consequences of 'lack of interest by officialdom and by educationalists in the mentally subnormal child' (op. cit.).

children (i.e. the parents of the children) that go to these training centres that are potty trained—that means they're a bit more intelligent—they're not so much trouble as these. It's us that need the most help that get the least.

Girl: 6 yrs. (pilot study)

Well, I think it would give me a break for half a day and I also think it's good for her to be with other people, because I feel the time will come when she'll have to go away into a home and I think this will gradually break her in.

Girl: 8 yrs. (pilot study)

They've got nothing like that round here, not for children like her. She's got these two to play with (siblings) but other than these, I mean, she's got nowhere to go, as you might say. She can't go and mix with other children and play on the streets like they can, she's got to rely on the others coming to her. I think if she was with a lot of children similar to herself she would see them trying to do things for themselves and she would try to do things for herself . . . she don't see nobody, it must be lonely for her.

Girl: 8 yrs.

I don't think the council are interested in them, myself, not in the children. I think they could do more for a day-centre for them. I know she can't be taught, but I think they should do *something* for them.

(Severe physical and mental handicap)

Boy: 6 yrs.

Well, to my mind . . . there seems to be a lapse up to 7 years old and I think they could do a little bit more. I mean, after they get to 5. I mean, you do the very best for your child, but I think in some cases . . . they could do a lot from 5 to 7 that they're missing. I think they could do with a bit more help. I mean, a qualified person can get a lot more out of a child than a mother can, because they know different ways to do a right thing. I mean, if they're left till 7, and I know children been left longer, well, they get more dependent on their parents and I think then they find the change harder.

Boy: 1 yr.

Well, I don't know—it just depends. If he's got to go amongst children that are badly handicapped, to be honest, I'd say No. I want him to go with children that are not too bad—I want him to go amongst children that can teach him, it's no use pushing him amongst children that are worse than himself, is it?

Boy: 7 yrs.

Not so long ago we had somebody, you know, to find out whether he was at school. And I thought 'Well, they've taken their time coming, like'. I mean, if it had been a normal child, they'd have been round more or less straight away.

Girl: 7 yrs.

Well, no, I don't really think I would. I can't see what they'd be able to do that we couldn't, with her. As you see, she sits like this all day and you really have to know how to give her a drink. I know it might sound funny, but you do have to know when she's going to open her mouth and that sort of thing. Well, I don't think strangers—'course they're not used to her—they wouldn't know. I don't think there are any centres for children like these.

Boy: 8 yrs. (Severe physical handicap)

All they go for is for the parents to have a rest—well, I think it's a wicked shame. I think they could do far more with them. They don't even seem to read to them or show them pictures or things like that. I mean, we do far more for them at home than what they're doing.

There is no doubt that standards of care offered at day-centres of all kinds need to be very high indeed to equal or improve on that provided by all but a very small minority of families, if the East Midlands sample is any criterion. But in spite of the fact that doubts are expressed by some, most mothers would welcome the *right* to send their children to properly run day-centres where they could be certain that the children were happy and well cared for and, most important of all, enjoying advantages that home, however good, cannot provide. As it is, parents feel that they have to fight for their children, in order to obtain for them the kind of care which it is universally agreed is essential both for the children and their families. One father who happened to be present during an interview put it like this:

This is a lot of the trouble with children of this type. If the parent is like me, damned awkward, then you get what you want and your child gets somewhere. But if you're the normal run of people who accept the fact that authority is authority and 'this must be done in a certain way and we accept patiently that we must wait'—then they get nowhere fast. There's only one way to get anywhere if you've got kiddies like Maureen and that's to bang on the table.

The situation in the East Midlands seems to be part of a wider failure to make provision for some groups of handicapped children throughout the country. To quote Professor Tizard once more, speaking of services provided in the London area, 'When we looked for gaps, for families which were not getting much help, or which appeared to be particularly hard done by, two groups stood out: the pre-school defective and his family; and the most severely handicapped of the older age group, namely those too handicapped to attend ordinary day training centres.'

To turn to a more positive aspect of the question of education for the handicapped, we found that for children of normal intelligence whose physical handicaps are not too great, the problems can be solved in ordinary primary schools, when teachers and local authorities are prepared to be flexible and helpful. The latter point is sometimes more important than the degree of handicap and we were given instances both of schools which had exercised their imagination to accommodate children with quite considerable physical disability, and of some where lack of imagination had made life more difficult than it need have been for children with minimal physical disabilities. Mothers realize that extra demands are made upon teachers when they are willing to include handicapped children and are very appreciative when the effort is made, as the following comment illustrates:

> The head mistress is most helpful. We're very fortunate. She's so willing to help. And when they have such a big and busy school—it's not just like a small village school—it's a big school, you see, and overcrowded. I really think it's most magnanimous of them. They really are splendid—I've been delighted.

This quotation refers to a 7-year-old boy who was going to the local primary school every afternoon and then staying on after school for individual tuition by a teacher who had formerly been his home-teacher. His mother stressed how much he had benefitted from contact with boys his own age—the one thing that home teaching cannot supply. He was taken to school in his wheel-chair—he could walk only with the help of a 'Rollator' walking aid—and was seen every three months by the school medical officer to make sure that he was still able to cope with this regime.

Not all mothers are as fortunate, and attempts to include their children in normal schools sometimes come to grief over such things as need for help in the toilet, or even in getting to the dining room for school lunches.

Thirty-two (26%) of the school age children in the East Midlands sample were attending ordinary primary schools (i.e. 18% of the whole sample). Twenty-six of these children were of normal intelligence and only one of these 26 was more than mildly physically handicapped. Of the remaining six children, 3 had been pronounced 'backward' but had been accepted by ordinary schools and one of these was only able to walk with a walking aid. The last 3 of this group were classified as of 'uncertain' mental status—one was 4 years old, attending the nursery class of a primary school; she had not had any tests or ascertainment. One had been uncooperative on testing and had been given the benefit of the doubt until he could be re-tested. The third had been tested twice by the local authority and assessed by the Spastics Society in London. His mother said she did not know the results of these tests, and she was not satisfied that at 8 years old he was going to school in the mornings only. He was on a waiting list for a residential school (although it was not clear whether this was a school run by the Spastics Society or not) but his mother was upset at the idea of his going away from home at 9 years old and would have preferred a special day-school for him.

Only one child in the sample who was over school age and of normal intelligence was not having some kind of tuition. This child was waiting for a place in a day-school for physically handicapped children. He had been allowed to attend a normal school for a short time while his sister had been at the same school, because she had been able to help him to go to the toilet. However, when his sister left the school, he too, had to leave because no other arrangements could be made to give him this help.

Reference back to Table 6.I will show how small a part special day-schools and home-teaching played in the lives of children with cerebral palsy in the East Midlands sample, 11% and 3% respectively of the school-age children in the sample receiving this kind of tuition, including one child in a special class in an ordinary school.

If suitable education at a day school or day training centre cannot be provided for a child, the possibility of boarding school or of residential care may arise. We asked the East Midland mothers whether their children were on waiting lists for residential schools at the time of interview. Only thirteen, that is 10%, of the school age children were waiting for places in residential schools, six of these in schools run by the Spastics Society. Five were waiting for places in Local Education Authority schools. In two cases there was some doubt about whether the children had actually been included in waiting lists for school places; their mothers had interpreted some discussion that had taken place with workers from the Spastics Society about the *possibility* of boarding school as meaning that the children were definitely on such lists. Thus, boarding school was to be a solution for only a few of the East Midlands sample of children.[1] Twelve of these 13 children were among those who were already having some kind of tuition—3 in ordinary schools, 2 as 'weekly boarders', 1 at junior training centre (this little boy had only recently been diagnosed as deaf and had been given a hearing aid at 5 years +), 1 at special school and 4 through home teachers. This means that for those *not* at school, there was not even the expectation of residential provision in the near future.

A further 14 children were actually on waiting lists for permanent care. Only 3 of these were attending junior training centres for 5 days a week. Five more were attending voluntary play-groups or day-centres for 1 or 2 days per week, and the remaining 6 were having no day-care at all. All but one of these children were already over 5 years old. Mothers made the point that to be sent away from home is harder for the children when they have not been used to spending even the day-time with people other than their families, and this certainly makes it harder for their parents to adjust to their going. Once more, it seems that the more disadvantages a child sets out with, the more will accrue to him as time goes on, unless much greater efforts are made to reverse this trend than is the case at present.

[1] Remembering here, of course, that some East Midlands children of this age group were already away at school or in residential care and so were excluded from the sample.

The existence of waiting lists is an indication that provision of residential care for severely mentally and physically handicapped children is not adequate to meet demand. The same is true of boarding school provision for less handicapped children who have been ascertained as educable but for whom suitable day-school provision is not available. However, the size of waiting lists is no indication of *potential* demand and, paradoxically, as Tizard has pointed out with respect to institutional care for the mentally subnormal, if more and better residential provision were to become available, a reserve of hidden demand would be revealed that would quickly overtake the new level of provision (op. cit.). The result could be even longer waiting lists, unless standards of community care should also improve to such an extent that stronger incentives were provided to keep children at home than to have them cared for in institutions, because 'the better the quality of institutional care, the less reluctance parents will have in parting with a child and the more readily they will be advised to do so.' The influence of social and economic factors on parental attitudes to such provision is probably important but as yet imperfectly understood.

We asked the mothers in the East Midlands sample if they would be willing to consider either boarding school, residential training centre, or residential care in a home of some kind that did not provide any kind of training or education. We also asked them whether they agreed with their husbands over this decision, thinking that this might be a potential source of conflict in these families. Taking this last point first, 146 (81 %) of the mothers reported that they were in agreement with their husbands over this issue, 17 (9 %) were not, and of the remainder, 5 mothers did not have husbands to consult about such decisions, 5 more did not know what their husbands thought as they had never discussed it, 4 had never thought about it at all, and in one instance, the interviewer failed to get a reply to the question.

Thirty-four (19%) of the sample agreed with their husbands that their children should not have any kind of residential care or education. As might be expected, the majority of these children (25) were only mildly physically handicapped and either or normal intelligence or educable in special day-schools. Only 5 mothers of severely physically handicapped children

said that they would not consider residential care of any kind—
4 of these children were also mentally handicapped, the fifth
had not been assessed (he was only 2 years old).

On the other hand, 58 parents were willing at least to *consider*
any kind of residential care as a possibility some time in the
future. Thirty-five of these had children with confirmed mental
defects, and 19 of these children were also severely physically
handicapped. A further 12 children in this group were severely
physically handicapped and of uncertain mental status. The
majority of these mothers recognized that they would not be
able to manage to care for their children as they grew older and
heavier, however much they might want to keep them at home.
The parents of the less handicapped in this group seemed to
share a common attitude of willingness to consider any course
of action that might broaden the experience of their children in
the future. What worries a great many parents is, that so many
of the institutions that care for the very handicapped seem to be
so far from the children's own homes that it is very hard to
keep in touch with them at all once they have gone away. The
problem is not quite so acute for the children who go to boarding schools where the holidays are long, frequent and regular.

A third group of 54 parents were willing to accept boarding
schools or training centres, but not permanent care which was
not related to education or training of some kind. These parents
seemed to make a sharp distinction between parting with their
children so that the children would benefit in an obvious way,
and 'sending them away'. Most of this group had children
whose physical handicaps were mild or moderate, only 13 of
them being severely physically handicapped. Most of this third
group of mothers had many doubts and reservations about
allowing their children to go away at all, and said that they
would only consider it if there were no other way of getting
something done for them.

A small group, 12 mothers out of the whole sample, had quite
positive attitudes to the idea of residential school or care and
thought that this was the best solution to the problem both for the
child himself and for the family as a whole, some of them because
they found the child was a source of disruption of family relationships, upsetting their husbands and the other children.

When the responses of the whole sample to these questions
are considered, there is a strong suggestion that the majority of

parents have realistic attitudes to the possibility that residential care may or may not be necessary or desirable for their children at some time. For example, 52 mothers out of 58 having severely handicapped children would be prepared to consider it if necessary. So were 71 mothers of the 77 children with known mental handicaps. (A considerable number of these were also among the children with severe physical handicaps, too, of course.) On the other hand, most of those mothers who would not consider such a step at all, feeling it to be unnecessary, had mildly handicapped children. There was some evidence to support Tizard's view (op. cit.) that there is 'a tendency for middle-class parents to seek hospital care more readily than do working-class parents'. Twenty-six, or 62%, of all the class I, II and III w.c. parents in the East Midlands sample were willing to consider any kind of residential care as opposed to 38 or 28% of those in class III m., IV and V.

The mothers' own words on this subject best demonstrate how they feel about it.

Girl: 6 yrs.

Yes, if I felt it would do her good, yes, definitely. I mean, I suppose she'll get used to it, like, but I would let her go, for her own good, later on. Not to 'ship her off', like . . .

Girl: 2 yrs.

If it wasn't going to retard her more. If it was going to help her, I would do anything and let her go anywhere . . . If I were confident that she were given (individual) attention I'd be very willing. In fact, I'd be reasonably relieved, to be quite honest, because then we could have other children, if she was going to a residential school. I rather—don't like the thought of her going to a residential mental hospital . . . because when she went to (a hospital for the mentally subnormal, for temporary care) they found it terribly difficult to manage her. In fact, my husband used to go and feed her quite often because they'd had this difficulty feeding her. Well, when my husband first went, she was left in her cot and it was sort of middle of the afternoon and she'd had her pyjamas on all day and she was just left lying in the cot.

Boy: 5 yrs.

You mean to board? No, because I think home life's important to him. I want him to go to school and I want him to go to school as soon as possible, but not to be away all the time, no.

Girl: 5 yrs.

I know it's a job to find places for them—I *do* know. I've often
wondered if there isn't places . . . places where they could go in
the week and come home weekends to us—you know—sort of
weekly places, weekly rents. I haven't heard of any. We don't
want her to go but it's something that's got to come eventually.

Boy: 7 yrs.

No, I don't want him to. No, because (his father) was left as a baby
and he's been brought up without a mother or a father, sort of
thing, and he'd never want one of his to go away . . . I don't
think he'd stop at a residential school, anyway, I think he'd fret,
I do, and that's not just being emotional myself. I know what he's
like.

Boy: 6 yrs.

Well, (my husband) used to think he should go away and I didn't.
We varied on that, you know. He said I'd been a bit too silly with
him because he said 'Matthew doesn't know, really.' (He didn't
know). 'Cos I always say a man hasn't got the love that a woman's
got for them. But I'm coming round, 'cos I'm getting fed up with
all the work, 'cos it's me all the time.

Boy: 6 yrs.

We've just been to see Professor —— and he told us that his brain
hasn't developed and he really ought to go in an institution, which
sounds dreadful to me. We don't like the idea very much at all,
but we've had to put his name down in case there comes a time we
can't cope.

Girl: 6 yrs.

Yes, she is on a waiting list, she's been on nearly three years now.
We were discussing this with Dr —— and he said he couldn't
promise any particular date but he more or less told us that it
wouldn't be for quite a few years from now . . . She doesn't miss
us and she's quite happy as long as she's being looked after so I
don't see as, psychologically, it's going to have any effect on her
to go to permanent care, even tomorrow. Now, with a child that's
very attached to its parents, the child should perhaps be older. And
then again I think it's a lot to do with the parents. Now, both my
husband and I quite frankly want her to go to permanent care—we
both agree. And I would agree with it if they came to me and said

she's got to go for permanent care next week. I mean, maybe I feel —and I think I would feel—a bit guilty about the fact that I do want her to go to permanent care, but I *do* feel this way.

Boy: 6 yrs.

No, we don't agree but we don't make a big issue of it. (My husband) has thought for the last few years that everything ought to be done to get him away, because they're *not* doing anything. Well, I think they are, it's just that there's so many people wanting places. My husband thinks that he is one of the cases that should be away. He thinks it affects the other children and home life having him here. Things are a lot happier when he isn't here and I realize that it would be better for him to go, but I've only just felt like this. At first I wouldn't have parted with him for anything, but I realized that you've got to make arrangements for these things a long while before they go. When he gets to 8 or 9 he will be impossible for me to handle.

Boy: 4 yrs.

Well, it all depends *why* he went. If he went to a residential school with the object in mind of training him to work and speak and that, provided he came home—I know he'd have to stay the term at school—provided he came home holidays and that, I wouldn't mind but I wouldn't put him away *as* put him *away*, if you understand. And of course if they tell me they didn't think he can go to school, he'll stop home. We won't part with him.

Girl: 5 yrs.

He (husband) don't want her to go away, you know, to school; but I say if she'll get better education away, it's best to go, isn't it, even if it's a long way away. But he doesn't agree with that. The nearest school is in Cumberland somewhere and it's such a long way to go, isn't it?

Boy: 2 yrs.

Never. No, he's not that handicapped that he wants putting in an institution. I mean, I can cope with it . . . I'd never let him go as residential. I believe a child is much better off in his own house.

Professor Tizard[1] has pointed to differences between the type of residential care provided by local authorities for normal children deprived of a normal home life, children, that is, 'in

[1] Op. cit.

care', and the type of residential care provided for mentally handicapped children. Parents, too, are aware of the short-comings of many institutions for the handicapped and know that these are not the right alternatives to home care should this become too difficult for them to provide. Howard R. Kelman[1] sums up the situation thus: 'The real problem is not whether institutional care *per se* is better (or worse) than home-rearing *per se* but rather whether care in a particular institution with a specific programme or home-care in a particular family environment (and for a specific time) will better meet the assessed needs of a particular child.'

[1] Op. cit.

CHAPTER 7

WHO WILL HELP?—THE FAMILY AND THE SOCIAL SERVICES, STATUTORY AND VOLUNTARY

It is important that the parents are given continuing casework support by experienced doctors and social workers throughout, but especially in the first few months and years.

MARY SHERIDAN[1]

As we have already seen, families with handicapped children lead lives which in many respects are very like those of families with only normal children. However, there is one way in which their lives are almost inevitably different—that is, in their need to have much more contact with the various social services than most families. We found, for example, that the majority of the East Midlands children (74%) had regular contact with consultants (mainly paediatricians), attending hospital outpatient departments at intervals ranging from one month to one year for this purpose. These routine visits often affect other members of the family and always present the mothers with something extra to be fitted into busy lives—father's role in this respect is usually negligible because he is at work, except when he takes time off to transport his wife, or when his shift coincides with a hospital appointment.

The existence of handicap also makes it likely that the family will become the concern of certain social work agencies, both voluntary and statutory, although this does not follow as inevitably as does contact with doctors. Spastic children who are also mentally handicapped become the responsibility of the mental welfare officer, who is employed by the local authority to help and advise both the mentally ill and the mentally subnormal who are living at home. School medical officers and

[1] Op. cit.

school welfare officers may visit the homes of children who are attending ordinary or special schools, to advise on questions relating to education. Again, school medical officers or psychologists may call to make assessments of the child's educability and special educational needs. Someone from the local authority's Welfare Department may visit to offer help with the problem of adapting ordinary homes to accommodate children who cannot manage steps, or, who can only be mobile in bulky wheelchairs—local authorities are empowered to make alterations to homes or to offer grants towards the cost of such alterations. Health visitor services are for the handicapped as much as for the normal. If the family has a child who is blind or deaf as well as physically handicapped, someone with a special responsibility for such children may visit as well. Voluntary bodies of all kinds offer services for people with specific handicaps, sometimes in cooperation with local authorities, sometimes independently. Thus, the fact of having a handicapped child means that one *can* become the focus of attention from all kinds of people who, but for that chance event, might never have been aware of one's existence.

The need for advice and counselling of parents who have a handicapped child is emphasized in all the literature on handicapped children, and we wanted to find out how much help of this kind had been made available to the East Midlands mothers and what they thought about it—in essence, a kind of consumer research. This sort of approach is always open to the criticism that mothers' recollections will be inaccurate and that the accounts that they give of events will be very different from those given by the professionals concerned. There is undoubtedly an element of truth in this. In any situation which involves two or more people, there are inevitably two or more ways of experiencing that situation. In the kinds of situation we are discussing here, the professional person, however well-intentioned, may fail to make his role and his intentions clear to the mother. So complex and variable are our social services, that the public is often confused by them. The proposals of the Seebohm Committee[1] are, in part, a recognition of this fact. However, unless or until the recommendations of the Seebohm Report are translated into action, the need is for social service personnel to explain again and again who they are and what

[1] Seebohm Report, op. cit.

help they can offer. At the present time, people can be uncertain of the identity of the person who visits them. They are not always sure which local authority department the visitor represents or what kind of help they are entitled to expect from such a visitor.[1]

The exception is the health visitor. She is clearly recognizable in her uniform[2] and is expected to be able to give practical advice on the 'right' way to tackle problems such as difficulties with feeding babies or getting them to sleep. Mothers also expect that she will approve of some of the things they do with their children and disapprove of others[3] and that her concern is mainly with the physical well-being of the child. This may not be the image that the modern health visitor would wish to project, but it is one which seems to persist in the minds of many mothers. From the mother's point of view, the function and role of, for example, the mental welfare officer is not nearly so well defined, nor is that of the visitor from the Spastics Society or some other voluntary body.

All such visitors are referred to in the East Midlands survey as social workers. This will not satisfy those who would prefer to confine this designation solely to those who have had a casework training intended to enable them to exercise special skills in the detection and resolution of personal as opposed to practical problems. From the point of view of the clients, how-ever, the difference is not one which is readily discernible, in respect of personnel or problems. Very few of the East Mid-lands mothers indicated that they appreciated the difference between the 'home visitors' from the Spastics Society Family Help Unit in Nottingham, who were not trained in casework techniques, and the Society's Regional Social Worker, who was. Both were simply from the Spastics Society. However, although the term 'social worker' is used in the text, it was not used at all in the questions put to the mothers.[4]

In the quotation at the beginning of this chapter, the medical profession, too, is seen by one of its most distinguished and experienced members as having an important social work role. As we have seen in Chapter 2, the way in which they approach

[1] One of the best guides through this labyrinth is *The Consumers' Guide to the British Social Services* by Phyllis Willmott—a Pelican Original, 1967.

[2] In some local authority areas uniform is no longer worn. In others, only the colour to be worn is specified, often the traditional navy-blue.

[3] See Newson, J. & E., 1963, op. cit. for evidence of mothers' attitudes to health visitors.

[4] See Appendix, III.

their difficult 'social work' tasks of breaking the news of handicap to the parents, and of initiating and maintaining a relationship with them that will facilitate further discussion on a helpful level, is not always successful from the mother's point of view. However, the views expressed there concerned the hospital consultants with whom the mothers had been in contact. The situation could be different in respect of general practitioners. We asked mothers how helpful they thought their family doctors had been with the handicapped child.

Twenty-five mothers (14% of the whole sample) said that they had found their family doctors helpful in specific ways. Specific help included regular monthly visits by the doctor to see the handicapped child at home although he had not been asked to call (in seven instances). Some doctors had contacted various local authority departments on behalf of the parents and had concerned themselves with attempts to obtain temporary or permanent care. Active interest of this kind is very much appreciated by parents, particularly as most of them think of general practitioners as being over-burdened with work; the doctor's special concern for the problems of the handicapped is thought of as being extra to the service that can normally be expected of him.

Seventy-five mothers (42%) said that they had found the family doctor helpful in a general sort of way although they could not think of any specific action he had taken. Far more often it was an attitude of understanding and helpfulness that had been conveyed to the mother, and a frequent comment in this context was that the doctor would always come when called to the handicapped child—as though some mothers half expected that he would not necessarily do so. Similarly, a doctor who will listen to mothers is valued very highly, even if he cannot actually do anything else. As with mothers' feelings about the helpfulness of consultants, their comments on helpful and unhelpful general practitioners seem to indicate that their perception of their relationship with their medical advisers is influenced very much by the doctor's ability to convey the idea that he is an ally, working *with* the parents, not against them. The sample was almost equally divided in its views on this matter, 56% finding their family doctors helpful and 44% not doing so. The comments that illustrate mothers' attitudes have been chosen so that this balance of views is retained.

Boy: 3 yrs.

Oh yes, yes. I don't think I should ever have got through without him. Well, everything I wanted to know, you know, he's tried to do his best for me. And he told me if I didn't let up at one time, where I would land up! I was getting a really—nervous wreck.

Boy: 2 yrs.

No, no help whatsoever. I went to him a few months back—I felt at screaming point with me own nerves and he said 'You'll find as he gets better, you'll unwind yourself and won't feel so tense.' He gave me nothing, no advice. I said, 'Is there anybody I can get in touch with about him?' I said, 'I've got to talk to somebody.' He said, 'I don't know anybody'. Didn't advise me or nothing. I mean, he *must* have known somebody I could have got in touch with.

(This mother later got in touch with the Spastics Society herself.)

Boy: 6 yrs.

My own doctor has been extremely good . . . He's one of these doctors who believes in coming every month, which he does do. He's extremely good, apart from help for Jonathan—something I feel *I* need something to boost me up, you know.

Boy: 3 yrs.

I never go and ask him for anything. I always think they'll say, 'Well, get out of it the same as you got into it.'

Girl: 6 yrs.

Yes, I think so—yes, he has . . . Let's put it this way, if there was nothing he *could* do, at least he has *tried* to do something for us and I think that means a lot.

Girl: 2 yrs.

No—but I think probably it's our own fault that he hasn't because we've never been to him, you see. I think with attending the hospital and having our drugs and everything from there, fortunately I haven't had to go to him at all and so therefore we haven't chatted—we did go once after we'd started going to the hospital and I must admit he did spend about half an hour talking to us about children like her—explaining to us about the attacks she had.

Boy: 4 yrs.

He simply is a doctor that . . . everyone seems to have the same opinion—you see, he seems to be writing out a prescription when you're walking in the surgery and he doesn't give you time to explain what's the matter and I feel a bit embarrassed going round —'cause I don't know how to approach him, you know. I'm not one for going to doctors.

Girl: 7 yrs.

Oh, he has, yes. Probably with her being as she is, he's probably rushed to see her. Up to having her, there was a barrier—you know, there's a barrier between the doctor and yourself, you sort of can't get over that barrier. Well, since I've had her, he's been more like a—well, more like a father, really. You could take any problem to him—that barrier's been . . .'

Boy: 3 yrs.

No, I wouldn't, far from it. Well, maybe I'm a bit touchy on the subject but I find that his attitude at times has been, 'Oh, that mother is not worth bothering about.' I don't think he understands these sort of children. It's difficult, really, to put a word to it but it's his attitude with Kenneth. He has a son practising in the same practice, now, and—of course, they're very busy—but *he* does find time to treat him normally, whereas the older one just looks at him—queer—you know.

Girl: 7 yrs.

I always ask doctor if I want to know anything. (Interviewer: Your own doctor?) Yes—I talk to him like talking to my Dad.

The medical profession itself is well aware that there are problems to be solved and that the acknowledged difficulty of communicating technical facts to lay people (and worried lay people at that) is a crucial one when it comes to establishing and maintaining a workable relationship with them. In an interesting discussion of the problem,[1] Dr T. A. Quilliam stresses the importance of the supportive role to be played by the general practitioner and points to two difficulties—first, that they may not 'possess the knowledge and experience to perform this task adequately' and second, that 'medical students are not instructed in the technique of communication with patients and those

[1] Quilliam, T. A. 'Clinical Communication—a Contemporary Problem.' *Med. Biol. Illust.*, **15**, 66–8, 1965.

practitioners who have learned to do so with truth, tact and sincerity have only done so by trial and error after much conscientious effort and soul-searching'. These comments were made with particular reference to congenital heart conditions and heart surgery for children, but they apply equally to other situations.

Communication is never a one-sided affair, of course. Dr Errington Ellis, discussing 'What the Doctor has to offer'[1], points out that 'Some parents are relaxed and friendly, skilled communicators and good witnesses. Others are not but it is important to meet them all and to listen to them, because they are an important part of the child's environment and their attitude to their child's disability is probably the most important factor in his life.'

Turning now to other social workers and their significance in the lives of the East Midlands families, we found that only 10 mothers said that they were not visited by anyone at all. One hundred and ten of the rest were visited by more than one agency, 75 by two, 33 by three and 2 by four. To take the health visitor first, with her nursing training followed by specialist training for her work with families, she seems on the face of it to be the ideal bridge between the medical world and parents bringing up handicapped children in their own homes. As a member of a local authority department and a key worker in the fields of preventive medicine and public health, which are the local authorities' main contributions to the National Health Service, she has a unique opportunity to act as a co-ordinating agency between the three branches[2] of the health service and other local authority services. She knows how the departments work, what services they offer and how to go about obtaining these services. She also has a better chance of knowing which families have a handicapped child because she knows of all the babies born in her area and has a duty to contact all new mothers. Some local authorities give individual health visitors special responsibility for particular groups—the handicapped, the elderly or the mentally ill, for example—but their main concern in most areas is with normal babies and young children

[1] Ellis, E. in *Teaching the Cerebral Palsied Child*. Ed. James Loring. Spastics Society, William Heinemann, 1965.

[2] i.e. The hospital service, the family doctor service and local authority health service. These three are administered separately from one another, although unification of health service administration is under discussion.

and their mothers. The number of handicapped children in the area looked after by any one health visitor will not be large, so that (like the general practitioner) she will not necessarily have the opportunity to become really familiar with the problems of managing such children at home. On the other hand, the fact that these children are few in number means that it should be possible for her to concentrate more of her time on them than on some of the well babies of experienced mothers who need her least.

We found that, according to mothers' reports, 75% of the 55 children who were under 5 years old were being visited by health visitors at the time of interview—40% of them 'regularly', i.e. 3 or more times a year and 35% 'occasionally', i.e. less than 3 times a year. Twelve of the 18 children who were 2 years old or less were being visited, 7 of them regularly. Most of these mothers had welcomed the health visitors and found them kind and helpful, in spite of the fact that they had been unable to solve particular difficulties: the mothers of children who were difficult to feed, for example, did not say that the health visitor had been able to offer any advice about this. A mother who wanted more advice about equipment for her child did not get it from the health visitor (or from anyone else). Some of the comments made by the mothers show that they do not really expect health visitors to be able to help them but that they appreciate the *intention* to help. Other comments show that some of them feel that the health visitors are avoiding them because they know that they will not be able to offer help and feel at a loss in the face of handicap.

Girl: 2 yrs.: first and only baby, very difficult to feed

'Oh, yes, yes, the health visitor; she's very nice, she is—it's the one I should see if I went to the clinic, you know. She comes to see why I haven't been—perhaps once in every 3 months. I think she comes to encourage me to go to the clinic, really, but she's very, very nice—you know—if she could help in any way I'm sure she would, and she's asked if I wanted anything.

Boy: 8 yrs.

They just don't know what to say to me. So—it isn't their fault. It's so rarely that they come across a child like this that they just don't know where to begin with them, really.

Boy: 2 yrs.

I don't know that health visitors are awfully well trained for this . . . I wouldn't dream of asking the health visitor because they've got too wide a field.

Girl: 2 yrs.

During the first 10 months of her life I expected her to come and I was longing to talk to somebody—or perhaps it was the first 6 months—I was absolutely longing to talk to somebody and every time she came up the road I thought 'Surely she's coming to see me this time.' Because I didn't know she was a spastic. She did all this screaming and nobody came anywhere near and . . . this probably put me against her (the health visitor) a little bit. I think she would be helpful if she could be helpful but—there's nothing much they can say. They don't seem to have a lot of experience in it and they just sympathize and say 'Yes, dear' and so on and I don't know that you feel a lot better for that . . . I don't suppose *she* would say that she knew a lot about it, if you asked her and therefore I don't have a lot of confidence in her . . . But I always welcome her—I welcome anybody—just breaks the monotony.

Boy: 6 yrs.

I couldn't tell you the last time she came. That does really—I *do* feel a bit upset about that. She did used to come odd occasions, but only very rare, never made a regular visit. It's 12 months since her —I've had plenty of help—I'm not grumbling—from other sources, but I do think that it wouldn't have hurt her to have called and seen how I was occasionally. I mean, if they can visit normal, healthy children, I'm sure they can come and just have a look at these, that's how I feel about it.

The health visitor's duty to the normal child ends when he starts school and becomes the responsibility of the school medical services. This usually happens at 5 years of âge—not many children attend state schools before that age. However, as we have seen, handicapped children are not always provided with appropriate education or day-care at the age of 5. More than a third of the East Midlands children who were 5 or older were not provided for in this way by local authorities and so were not benefiting from school health services, 46 children in all. Of these, 37 were known to have some degree of intellectual impairment. As we said at the beginning of this chapter, the responsibility for the welfare of mentally handicapped children lies with the local authority Health Departments who employ mental welfare officers to visit the children and their families at home. Where the children are attending local authority day-centres or special care units, they are constantly under the supervision of the local authority or the hospital service and it might be argued that in these circumstances there is less need for the family to be visited by the mental welfare officer. Where the children are not being provided with day-care, both for the child and the family, the need for the advice and support of the mental welfare officer seems *prima facie* to be greater. In the East Midlands sample, the priorities appeared to have been reversed. Of the 18 mentally handicapped children who were aged 5 or over and who were attending day-centres, 16 were also being visited by the mental welfare officer. Of the 37 who were not attending day-centres, again 16 were being visited by mental welfare officers, 11 of the remainder were sometimes seen by the health visitor (often because there were younger children in the family) and 10 were visited by neither the mental welfare officer nor the health visitor.

This might be an area where health visitors could be of great service, continuing to keep in touch with the children who are not in schools or day-centres after the age of 5, particularly in those instances where no other local authority social worker is in regular contact with the family. The concept of community care for the handicapped must seem to be no more than a bad joke to families such as these unless somebody translates the idea into practical action. Life is particularly hard for mothers caring for physically and mentally handicapped children if no day-care is provided for them, and it would appear to make sense to divert scarce social worker services from the families who already benefit from this day-time relief to those who do not.

As we have seen, mothers realize that the health visitor does not normally have special knowledge of handicap and are consequently not surprised when she is unable to offer specific advice or help. The mental welfare officers, on the other hand, do have a special field and could, perhaps, more confidently be expected to have some expertise to offer to mentally handicapped children and their families. In practice, this did not seem to be so for the East Midlands children. Unless the mental welfare officer had been instrumental in helping parents to get either day-care or residential care for the children, the opinion of the mothers in many cases seemed to be that he was as little able as the health visitor to help in managing the child at home. This is not really surprising. There is a chronic shortage of workers in the field of mental health, relatively few of such workers as there are have professional social work qualifications and the distribution of trained workers is uneven throughout local authority areas.[1] In these circumstances, home visits must be less frequent than is desirable (15 families were visited by mental welfare officers three or more times per year, 26 twice per year or less) and continuing casework support cannot be possible. It is arguable whether all, or even most, families are in need of such support, particularly if adequate day-care is provided. The comments that follow all refer to mental welfare officers.

Boy: 6 yrs. 11 mths. No local authority day-care

Well, he doesn't have much to say. He just wants to know if there's anything he can do in any way to help, which he can't and that's about all that goes on.

Boy: 5 yrs. No local authority day-care. Family recently moved

But of course, there's nothing they could do—it's a waste of time. *You* knew there was nothing they could do and *they* knew there was nothing they could do. They just walked in—'How is he?'—and went again. I think they upset you more than anything.

Boy: 6 yrs. No local authority day-care

They would help, but I honestly can't see what they can do for him, you know. But it is through the help of the health officer that we hope we've got him in this training centre.

Boy: 6 yrs. Special care unit for 6 days per week

The mental health officer—he came and it was him that got him into this day-care, you see. But, I mean, apart from that I've not really got any problems with him at home. He's not really a big problem . . . I don't *count* him as a problem.

Girl: 7 yrs. No local authority day-care

Oh, he's only a very young man. He's very helpful—anything you ask. But of course, they're not doctors. He's very good but it's not like dealing with anyone that's medically—that knows about these things.

[1] Seebohm Report, op. cit.

The health visitors and the mental welfare officers are the local authority workers most likely to be in relatively frequent contact with families where there is a handicapped child. School medical officers or medical officers of health may make isolated visits for specific purposes—to make assessments of need for special education, for example, or for routine medical examination of children returning to special schools after the holidays—but these are not social work visits. The most highly specialized of the visitors to the families of cerebral palsied children are those employed by the Spastics Society itself. At the time the East Midlands survey was carried out, a 'home-visiting' service was in operation, using the Family Help Unit in Nottingham as its base. A more 'casework'-oriented service was then in the process of being set up and some mothers had been visited both by home visitors and by a social worker with a specific social work training. As we have already pointed out, the distinction between the two kinds of workers and the help they could offer did not seem to be apparent to the mothers concerned. When they were able to remember the names of the workers who had been to see them, it was possible to be sure that casework support had been offered to them, but not otherwise. All such visits have therefore been counted together. Twenty-six families had been visited 3 or more times in one year, and 126 once or twice in a year (83% of the sample altogether). Thus, more mothers had seen someone from the Society than from any other single agency. The part played by other voluntary bodies of all kinds was a very minor one. Only 18 mothers (10% of the sample) had visitors from these, mostly infrequent. The voluntary bodies concerned included the churches (11 mothers), mainly represented by vicars and priests, the National Society for Mentally Handicapped Children (2) Dr. Barnado's Homes (1), voluntary worker for a local group of the Spastics Society (1), voluntary worker for the deaf (1) and for the blind (1) (identity of organizations uncertain). One mother had been visited by someone concerned with running a weekly play-group for handicapped children.

The sample was almost equally divided into those who thought they were members, or were sure they were members, of local groups of the Spastics Society (91) and those who were not (89). There was doubt in the minds of some of the mothers about what it meant to be a member.[1] When mothers said they

[1] See Appendix I for an account of the structure of the Spastics Society.

were not sure, they were asked whether they paid a subscription to the local group or not. If they replied that they did, they were counted as belonging to the group, even if they took no part in its activities. The Spastics Society and its visitors make no distinction between members and non-members. The same help is available for all. Mothers had heard about the Society from a variety of sources. These are listed in Table 7.I.

TABLE 7.I

Mother's sources of information about the Spastics Society	No. of mothers
Consultant	29
General Practitioner	2
Physiotherapist	30
Almoner	1
Other parents or friends	18
Parents made contact on their own initiative	8
Spastics Society made first contact with parents	55
No contact	6
Other sources	31
	180

Comments on the helpfulness of visits by the Society's workers varied as did those on other kinds of visitors. Mothers hope that visitors will be able to give them advice about practical problems of management, about equipment and gadgets as these become available, about other sorts of help, such as short-term care. In some cases, they simply like someone to talk to who understands their problems, particularly in the earliest months of realizing that they have a handicapped child. A very basic need exists for more information of all kinds, both about the condition itself and about ways to meet the difficulties that arise from it. Until the recent publication of the book by Nancie Finnie,[1] there were few sources of specific advice which would be of real use to a mother with a child who was difficult to bath, change, feed and dress or could not be persuaded to sleep. The Spastics Society has published a small number of helpful pamphlets but these had found their way to only a few of the East Midlands mothers. Spastics News did not always reach

[1] Op. cit.

even those who belonged to local groups. Table 7.II lists the various channels through which mothers had obtained information about cerebral palsy.

TABLE 7.II

Sources of information about cerebral palsy	No. of mothers
Pamphlets or leaflets seen at hospitals	9
Spastics Society publications sent for by mothers	21
Spastics Society publications obtained via local groups	28
Books obtained from libraries	30
Books bought	17
Articles in the press, in magazines	69
Programmes on television and radio (particularly Women's Hour)	127
Other	25
None	11

NOTE: These figures do not add up to 180 because sometimes individual mothers had several sources of information.

It seems that relatively few mothers will turn to the printed word for information unless this becomes more readily available. One way to make certain that useful books and pamphlets actually reach the mothers would be for health visitors and social work visitors of all kinds to have these always available. They could then look *with* the mothers for solutions to particular problems and actually participate in applying suggested remedies or techniques to the difficulties of specific children. This would also help to meet the criticism made by some mothers, that social workers cannot help them because they lack practical everyday experience of handicapped children.

A difficulty arises if the kind of help which the family needs cannot be supplied by the worker, however resourceful he or she may be. This is inevitably the case when mothers would like good day-care for their children but there is no suitable provision available for them. The same is true when the temporary care that is available is of a kind that causes mothers to be wary of accepting it for their children, however much they may need the relief it affords. In this situation of scarce and inadequate provision, which applies particularly to the mentally handicapped who also have physical handicaps, the case worker is in a very difficult position. Faced with a family who are suffering strain because the community services are inadequate to meet their practical needs, how can he or she approach them? The concept of supportive casework relationships, which has its origins in psychiatry, is surely inappropriate when the family is in distress, not through any inherent weakness in its relationships, but rather because it is being forced to function in circumstances which would test any family. How many of the 'anxious', 'aggressive' and 'possessive' parents, described by psychologists and doctors as 'rationalizing' their need to 'get rid of' their children when they attempt to obtain residential education or care, would simply 'disappear' if both day and residential care were equally good and freely available? If choice of provision were a reality, as it is for those parents of normal children who can afford to educate their children privately, would such adverse value judgments of parental motives be made? It seems unlikely—parents who send their children to public schools are seldom categorized in these ways.

There are some parents, however, who very much appreciate the fact that someone is interested enough in their children to call and see them. They find this expression of society's awareness of their problem sufficient justification for such visits, even if no practical help can result. No mothers said that they had asked any worker not to call again, however disparaging they had been of the usefulness of visiting.

Two mothers expressed views that were hostile to the idea of supportive visits that had no practical outcome. They were both in need of practical help with a variety of problems. One also had personal problems, and was very much in need of day-time relief from her badly handicapped child, aged 6. A visitor had promised to see if this could be arranged but she had heard no more about it. Naturally enough, she felt she had been let down. The other mother felt there could be no point in having visitors who 'only asked a lot of silly questions'.

There were 32 mothers (18% of the sample) who had no strong feelings about social work visits. They were not hostile to them, but it seemed to make no difference whether any one visited them or not. Twenty-seven of them said that they would not like to be visited more frequently. Five said that they would always welcome anyone who called but that they did not *need* more visiting. Twenty-seven of these 32 mothers had mildly physically handicapped children and only 9 had children with known mental handicaps.

The rest of the mothers were either welcoming to social workers without reservation (52%) or gave them a qualified welcome (23%)—this last meaning that they made comments on the failure of the visits to have any useful outcome but that they welcomed the visitors just the same.

When we asked mothers whether they would like to be visited more often, almost 70% of them replied that they would not (123 mothers). Fifty-seven mothers felt that they would like to be visited more often. Of this group, proportionally twice as many had children whose mental status had been classified (by us) as uncertain (36%–21/58) or who were known to be mentally handicapped to some degree (36%–28/77), as had children who were known to be of normal intelligence (18%–8/45). Forty-eight of the mentally handicapped and unclassified children had no day-care or had only voluntary day-care provision for one or two days per week. It is therefore not surprising that their mothers should feel that they need more contact with possible sources of help. We have already seen that those having no day-care were less likely to be visited by mental welfare officers than those who were at a junior training centre (p. 164 of this chapter). The mothers who would like more social work support thus include some of those who pose the problem for caseworkers that we have discussed above. Is this, perhaps, the reason why they are visited less frequently than they would like?

We asked mothers the question, 'If you needed help or advice, who would you turn to first?', thinking that their replies would reflect to some extent the importance to them of the various social service and social work agencies. The distribution of their replies is given in Table 7.111.

More mothers thought that they would turn to the Spastics Society than any other agency (32%). Often this meant that they would contact the Family Help Unit in Nottingham to ask for emergency care, but sometimes secretaries of local groups of the Society were mentioned, too. Second in popularity were the general practitioners (16%). Local authority agencies, which included health visitors, mental welfare officers and the children's department (once) came third (12%). Consultants and physiotherapists accounted for 18% of choices between them

TABLE 7.III

To whom mothers of spastic children would turn first for help

Spastic Society	Spastics Society	Other vol. body	Own G.P.	Consultant	School	Physio-therapist	Hosp. almoner	L.A. agency	D/K	Other	Total
Members	37	—	13	7	1	8	—	11	12	2	91
Non-members	21	1	15	11	2	6	—	11	10	12	89
Total	58	1	28	18	3	14	—	22*	22	14†	180

* In 9 instances, this means the mental welfare officer.

† 'Other' includes family and friends, a school headmaster, a teacher of the deaf, a maternal and child welfare clinic and a school medical officer.

and when it is remembered that almost 80% of all the children in the sample were attending hospital out-patient departments, it is remarkable that no one considered the hospital almoner or medical social worker to be the source of help that would spring to mind first.

The information supplied by the East Midland mothers appears to lend some support to the case for a single social service department to whom all handicapped children and adults would be entitled to turn. However, unless such a department were able to tap greater resources than are at present available, the end result from the point of view of the public whom it would serve would not be any different. If provision of services is basically inadequate, rationalizing the channels through which such services can be obtained will not affect the outcome. On the other hand, if the social workers who are detecting need are also part of the department which will supply those needs, it is possible that a greater sense of urgency will be generated, and it will not be possible to lay responsibility for failure and delay at other departments' doors. The exception here will be the provision of education and training which would lie outside the province of such a department.

CHAPTER 8

SOME SPECIAL PROBLEMS

Bringing up any family involves coping with problems and making decisions that affect the welfare of the whole family. The presence of a handicapped child means both that some decisions are harder to make and that some arise that might not have had to be faced at all if all the children had been normal.

Three family problems seemed to us to be important, three kinds of decision-taking that would be complicated by, or arise from, the presence of handicap. First, and very basic, is the question of whether to have more children after the arrival of the cerebral palsied child. How to attempt to 'space' or 'plan' their children is something that concerns most parents, but it is of greater significance in families where there is a handicapped member. There are two main reasons for this. The management of a new baby added to the work involved with caring for the handicapped child may seem to the mother to be more than she can cope with. This can be so, even when the handicapped child is the only child. In one sense, mothers of more than one child have an advantage here, because they already know that they can manage an enormous amount of work and so may have greater confidence in their ability to carry any extra burden that is thrust upon them. Nevertheless, the presence of a child who will always need a great deal of care inevitably complicates the situation. In addition to this, almost all parents wonder whether they are likely to have another handicapped child. This worries some parents more than others, but it is unusual for the thought never to enter the mother's head, particularly when she is pregnant.

A second kind of decision more likely to arise where there is handicap, is whether to try to find other doctors or other forms of treatment for the child if that currently offered seems less than adequate.

The third kind of problem concerns the future of the child as he grows up. A decision may have to be taken about accepting or rejecting institutional care. Plans may have to be made to provide for a child who will never be able to compete in the open market for employment. All these decisions are influenced to a certain extent by the quality of the help available to the family and by the family's own resources.

We turn now to the question of having more children. We asked the East Midlands mothers three questions about this subject, in order to discover (i) their own feelings about having more children, (ii) whether they had had the opportunity to discuss the problem with medical advisers, and (iii) whether they had had any advice about methods of birth control.[1]

As might be expected, those mothers who had very lightly handicapped children were less troubled by this question than those with severely handicapped children. Considerations other than the handicap were important in some families, too. Some mothers hoped they had completed their families, having achieved the number of children they had planned for. One had reached the menopause soon after the handicapped child had been born. Some mothers had already become pregnant again before they knew about the handicap and 4 of the children had been adopted or fostered. Including all these mothers, half the sample (92) said that their feelings about having more children had not been changed by the arrival of the handicapped child. Another 3 had had another child *because* one was handicapped. Sixteen mothers had had another child although they would have preferred not to, and 61 (34%), including these 16, felt that they had been deterred from deliberately having more children. The three quotations which follow illustrate three very different ways of thinking about the problem.

Girl: 2 yrs. (Only child. A second baby was stillborn)

We asked (the paediatrician) if it could possibly happen again if we had more children. He said this was an absolute isolated case, that No, it couldn't happen again. I did speak to (the obstetrician) and he said, 'As soon as you're pregnant again, come to me'. And I said, 'Well, do you advise me to have any more, it having happened twice?' 'Oh, of course, dear, yes', he said. 'I'll do my best to see it should be all right next time. And next time I won't "farm you out". You'll be completely under me.' . . . I adore children. I'd love more children now, but I haven't a clue how

[1] See Appendix III.

we'd cope with it. This is why we sent for (social worker) last time, because we'd decided we wanted more children but how could we cope with them? We *could* cope with them, but—excuse the expression—it would be just a hell of a life. It's hard enough now. It's not very happy. It's an absolute nightmare, in fact. But we feel it would be worse. And yet it seems wrong that we should deprive ourselves when we both adore children. We wanted to talk this over with her—what sort of help we would need, ideally, and so on, and we rather came to the conclusion that it would all be rather costly—and that we couldn't come to any very satisfactory decision—and we're still thinking about whether to sell the house and go into something smaller so that we might be able to afford to have help; we certainly couldn't afford to in this house. Then again, we think, why go into a smaller house when what we really need is a bungalow. So we still haven't decided. It all boils down to cost, I think. (Interviewer: What suggestion did the social worker have?) She came to the conclusion that while I was carrying the baby, during the last few months and the first few months after the baby was born, I could do with living-in help. She also thought that I ought to have a chat with the obstetrician but he isn't the chatting sort. I rather object to throwing about five guineas down the drain to have a talk that he won't—I feel he won't want to talk this over. Although she thought I ought to do. Certainly I wouldn't hesitate to have a private consultation with him if I thought it was worth it and if I thought he was going to talk to me—when anyone tries to talk to him, he won't. The sister's almost sort of apologetic for you, that you should *dare* to address such a person. And also she thought that for some considerable time—and I thought, too—that *after* that I would need help in the house or with the children, but it all came down to the fact that it was all too costly. So we still haven't done anything.

Boy: 6 yrs. (*First child of three*)

I just think it's essential to have more children when you have a handicapped child.

Boy: 6 yrs. (*Only child*)

Yes, they (the doctors) all seem to think it's a good idea—if not to have one of your own, to adopt one. But apparently to adopt one we should have to push Jeremy out, which seems to me a shame— push your own out for someone else's.[1] And I would very much like another one but my husband—no. We've ruined three lives,

---

[1] One other mother had been told this, too, but a third, whose children were all adopted, had no difficulty in adopting another when she discovered that the second adopted child was handicapped.

as far as he's concerned, and another one will always have Jeremy round it—providing it was normal, of course—I think there's a good chance that it wouldn't be, and he says he just couldn't cope with another one like that—it would be too heart-breaking.

No one can tell a mother what she should do about this problem. All a doctor can do, if he is sufficiently well-informed, is to discuss with the mother the probability that history will or will not be repeated in her case, so that she can make the decision herself. This kind of discussion, genetic counselling, useful and important as it is, has an inherent difficulty that has to be faced by parents and advisers alike. This difficulty is, that the usefulness of such counselling depends on the parents having understood the concept of probability and its relevance to their dilemma. For some conditions, the probability that a mother of a handicapped child will have a second child with similar handicaps can be stated with some accuracy. Spina bifida is one, and for this condition recurrence rates have been calculated on reliable data. However, although it is possible to say with confidence that, of all mothers of children with spina bifida, 1 in 15 will have another child with the same condition,[1] no one can say which individual mothers will fulfill the prediction.

This may not always be the case, however. According to a recent press report,[2] some results of research into conditions with a known genetic origin may have important consequences for the future development of genetic counselling. The report states that a technique has been evolved, whereby a sample of the unborn baby's cells may be obtained from the amniotic fluid which surrounds it. Laboratory tests can show whether there are abnormal chromosomes present in these cells. If there are, the doctor can know for certain that the baby will not develop normally, the pregnancy can be terminated and the mother can try again. The report refers particularly to the use of this test to detect mongolism (Down's syndrome), but indicates that in time it might be extended to other inherited diseases.

The technique described is still in its experimental stages. Some time in the future it may become a routine screening device for mothers who are known to have a family history of

[1] Hare *et al.* 'Spina Bifida Cystica and Family Stress.' *British Medical Journal*, September, 1966.
[2] *The Observer*, February 9, 1969.

genetic disorder, or for mothers who are over 40 years old and therefore statistically more likely to have a mongol child than are younger mothers. Before this could happen, special laboratories with trained personnel would have to be established.

With cerebral palsy, there is not even a recurrence rate to be taken into account. As yet, there is no clear evidence of an important genetic component in the causation of the majority of the conditions which are included under this heading.[1]

Of the 180 mothers in the East Midlands sample, none had had a second cerebral palsied child at the time of interview. One had had a child who had died during her second year, and this child had been blind and physically handicapped, although the mother did not say that her condition had been called cerebral palsy. The second child was normal and the third was the child in our sample.

The replies to our question asking mothers whether they had discussed this difficult problem with anyone are given in Table 8.I. Thirty-nine replied that they had never done so with anyone at all, neither professional people nor husbands, nor other relatives. These 39 included mothers from all social classes and their children had all degrees of mental and physical handicaps.

As one might expect, the kind and quality of advice varied with the adviser. Referring again to Professor Illingworth's discussion of the problem, we find that he suggests that what is known 'should be sufficient to make one cautious about promising parents of a child with cerebral palsy that another child will not be affected. A careful family history should be taken, and a cautious statement should then be made, explaining that it is unlikely that another child will be affected, but that the risk is very slightly greater than it is for others.' According to the East Midlands mothers, the advice sometimes given lacks the neces-

---

[1] *Illingworth* (op. cit.) gives kernicterus (i.e. the neurological damage that can result from Rhesus incompatibility and the haemolytic disease of the new-born that can follow this) as the main 'hereditary' type of cerebral palsy, accounting for 10% of all cases. It is now preventable by exchange transfusion and so should largely disappear. He goes on to review a variety of familial forms of cerebral palsy some of which he describes as 'sporadic'. *Denhoff* (op. cit., 1960) stated that 'cerebral palsy has its origin in hereditary factors in at least 10% of cases and probably more.' He listed several neurological conditions as instances of cerebral palsy associated with genetic factors. However, in 'Cerebral Palsy—its Individual and Community Problems' (ed. Cruickshank), 1966, Denhoff lists these same conditions and three others as being 'genetic neurological disorders which *simulate* cerebral palsy' (our italics). This seems to suggest that they are no longer considered to be cerebral palsies of genetic origin.

TABLE 8.1

Incidence of discussion on whether to have more children
and who discussed it with mother

Discussion with	No. of mothers
General practitioner	47
General practitioner and gynaecologist/obstetrician	4
General practitioner and pediatrician	7
General practitioner and both above	2
Gynaecologist/obstetrician only	6
Paediatrician	16
	82
Husband*	101
Friends/relatives	8
Others	14
No one	39

* This figure includes those who specifically mentioned their husbands. In some families the children just seemed to come along without the parents ever discussing it. In others the circumstances were such that no discussion was necessary.

sary caution, and the carelessly given injunction to 'go away and have another' is not always welcome. As one mother said:

> Oh, yes, he (the paediatrician) told us to go and have another straight away. I asked him if he'd got any. He said 'Yes'. I said, 'Are yours perfect?' He said, 'Yes'. I said, 'Well, you don't know what it's like, then, do you?' Because we'd had one stillborn and then we'd had Edna (the cerebral palsied child). That was two, and I thought that was enough.

This mother was not given any advice about birth control. However, our next quotation shows how much variation there can be in individual responses to similar situations. The mother speaking in this case had a great deal to deter her from having more children; she had been advised not to do so, but had chosen to ignore this advice. She was seen during the pilot stage of the study, and described how dangerously ill she had been during her pregnancy with the cerebral palsied child. She went on to say:

> When I knew I was going to have Felicity (2nd child), I was worried, because they told me if I had any more I could lose my life ... if it happened again there would be nothing at all they

could do for me. And they said the baby might live and be worse than what Vincent is now. But I thought, 'Oh, well, other folks risk it. If you take notice of them (the doctors) you'd never have any.' I've always said I'd like four and I'm intending to have four.

When she was seen she already had a normal little girl and was expecting another baby shortly. Her case illustrates the fact that it is impossible for a doctor to make an absolutely positive statement about the future. He can only suggest what might happen on the basis of his knowledge of the past. The actual decision must be taken by the mother herself.

There are many different aspects of the problem to be considered when a deliberate decision has to be taken—things are much easier in some ways when the matter is taken out of the parents' hands, and another baby arrives 'by accident'. This is particularly true when the handicapped child is the first baby and the management problems have been very great. This was the experience of the mother who speaks now:

> I think when you've had one like this, it's not the question of— that you'd get another one *like* her—it's just—how are you going to manage?... I don't think anyone could have been more against having another baby than me—I mean, I definitely didn't want any more, but of course he came along, and we're quite happy ... I didn't really want another one but I'm really glad I did, now. You don't realize what you've missed if you don't.

This sense of having 'missed' something is also expressed by the next mother and she indicates that she would welcome some positive encouragement to have another child. When asked whether her own family doctor had discussed this with her, she said:

> No, he hasn't—but he has said that we ought to get another one. I'm afraid he's never got time to sit and talk—he's always in and out. I sometimes feel I wish he would if it was only to back me up —you know. I feel that I want another one; I feel I want someone to give me a push. I had a word with (the paediatrician) last week about it and she said it would be a good thing ... I think—there are times—when I feel I've cheated (my husband) in not giving him a normal child—I sometimes feel I'm not being fair to him not to have another one.

We have noted elsewhere[1] that there was a higher proportion of 'only' children in the East Midlands sample than in the

---

[1] Chapter 1, p. 17.

normal 4-year-old sample (17% as opposed to 11%). Before drawing the conclusion that this is entirely due to the reluctance of mothers to have more children when the first is handicapped, we should take a closer look at the mothers and children making up the proportion of 17%, first discounting the 7 children who were 3 years old or less, because it is not unusual to find this interval between children in any family.

First, taking the 20 children of the East Midlands sample who were 4 years old at the time of interview, we find that 2, or 10% of them, are 'only' children. However, the number of children of this age in the sample is too small for this to have significance in itself. Of the 125 children aged between 5 and 8 years old, 22 (between 17% and 18%) are only children. This compares with 6% of the normal sample at the 7-year-old stage.[1] However, of this 22, 7 mothers had great difficulty in conceiving at all, 2 more had adopted or fostered the child, 2 were separated or divorced and another was expecting a second child. Thus there were reasons other than the birth of the handicapped child which could have been sufficient to account for its being a singleton.[2] Ten mothers only, of the 22, gave fear of having another handicapped child as the only reason for wishing to avoid becoming pregnant again (6% of the whole sample). Only one of these 10 mothers said that she had been to a family planning clinic for advice.

So far, we have been talking about mothers' discussing the advisability of having more children. Advice about methods of contraception appears to follow logically from such discussion, but it did not seem to have done so in practice, for most of the East Midlands mothers. It became clear during the pilot stage of the survey that this was a difficult subject to discuss for some mothers. To some it was embarrassing, and to others the relevance of detailed questioning was not apparent. For these reasons, when mothers simply answered 'yes' or 'no' to the question 'Did you do anything about birth control?' there was no more probing, except a question to attempt to confirm whether the mother had attended a birth control clinic, or had any other expert advice. Some replies, therefore, had to remain somewhat ambiguous and it is doubtful that the answer 'No'

[1] Newson, J. & E. In preparation.
[2] We do not have any information about the mothers in the normal-child sample on this point.

in this context means that nothing at all was done, since many of the mothers who replied in this way had been successful in limiting their families. It is more likely that these mothers meant that no advice had been sought, or that no mechanical or chemical contraceptive techniques had been employed. However, even making these reservations, it seems clear from Table 8.II that only a small proportion of the East Midlands mothers had had any expert advice about methods of birth control.

TABLE 8.II

Action on birth control

Mothers' action on birth control	Number
Family planning clinic	8
Sterilization	7
The 'pill'	18
Unspecified method	32
None*	82
Interviewer uncertain	2
Not applicable	14
Other	17
	180

* See text for reservations regarding this category.

The experience of the 61 mothers who felt discouraged from having more children was very similar to that of the whole sample in this respect. There was no evidence that they were more likely than the others to receive expert help. Sixteen of them had had one more child after the cerebral palsied child, and one had had two more, at the time of interview.

As we have said, mothers were diffident about discussing this subject with the interviewer and appeared to have been so with their doctors and other professional advisers. More surprisingly, the professionals, too, had been slow to suggest attending clinics or to give advice themselves, judging by the infrequency with which mothers mentioned such advice.[1]

This subject is now discussed openly in the press and on television. The local authorities have recently been empowered to set up advisory clinics within the National Health Service. In

[1] Hare *et al.*, reported similar findings—op. cit.

these circumstances, reticence seems out of place, and it would be very helpful if doctors and others who come into contact with mothers, could at least make sure that they are aware of the possibilities of getting advice, of what they could expect to happen to them if they went to a clinic, and of how much it would be likely to cost. One mother who had asked for 'the pill', for example, had been advised against it by her family doctor, because her own health was not good. She had decided not to go to the birth control clinic, as the doctor advised, because she thought the cost would be too high. Another had heard by chance from a friend that there were such things as clinics. She had thought, until then, that she had to consult her family doctor about these matters and as he was a Roman Catholic, had thought it would not be worth while to do so. Misconceptions of this kind could be avoided if doctors and social workers broached this subject themselves, and at least made sure that mothers knew sufficient about the kinds of help available to enable them to decide what to do.

We turn now to the second specific kind of decision we have mentioned—whether to seek private medical advice or treatment for a handicapped child. There are often comments in the literature on handicap about the frequency with which parents 'shop around', looking for miracle cures or more hopeful prognoses. Dr John Kershaw,[1] for example, speaking of advances in medical and surgical techniques, goes on to say:

> These advances, however, are not spectacular in the sense of offering splendid prospects to large numbers of the handicapped. They have even had unhappy consequences in that they have encouraged parents who had no grounds for hope to go on searching and to postpone the moment of truth in which they accepted their child as he was and began to set his feet purposefully on the right, though stony and uphill track. For most handicapped children that moment does finally come. It is a difficult but essential part of the duty of those who have to advise the parents to cut as short as possible the wearying and delaying round of visits to this hospital after that, to doctor after doctor and then down the ranks of the quacks and charlatans and even to country after country in search of the miracle; the longer the journey in search of the miraculous light the deeper the plunge into the final abyss of darkness.

[1] Kershaw, John D.: op. cit.

These things happen when the disability is one which openly proclaims itself in the first days or, at any rate, weeks of life. The position is similar yet different in the case of those disabilities which, though congenital, are not obvious early in life. A moderate degree of mental subnormality may not be suspected even by the family doctor or the health visitor until the child is five or six months old and even then they may be sufficiently uncertain to be reluctant to call the parents' attention to the possibility. Such a child *looks* perfectly normal and it is probable that not until he is reaching the end of his first year will the mother admit to herself that he is in any way backward. She, too, is likely to start on the weary round of the hospitals and consulting rooms, hoping to find someone who will tell her that all is well, and she may not be ready to face the facts until the child is nearing school age or even until his first weeks in school produce the practical proof that something is wrong. By this time, again, a pattern of over-protectiveness has been set and the future has been made a little more difficult.

Bice[1] states that although parents *may* be satisfied with the original diagnosis and advice and so feel no need to seek other advice, 'that is not the usual experience'. Denhoff and Holden[2] refer to 'shopping around' as the dangerous second stage of parental reaction to learning the truth about their child's condition. When mothers in the East Midlands sample were asked whether they had ever sought advice or treatment other than that provided by the National Health Service, 144 (80%) replied that they had never done so. The kinds of contact made by the remaining 36 (20%) are set out in Table 8.III, classified by social class.

TABLE 8.III

Treatment or advice sought outside the National Health Service

Social class	Faith healer	Lourdes	Private assessment or specialist consultation	Private physio-therapist	Osteo-path	Other	No. of mothers	Percentage of social class
I, II and III w.c.	3	0	5	0	2	1	10	24%
III man., IV and V	7	4	4	5	2	6	26	19%

[1] Bice, H. V. in *Cerebral Palsy—its Individual and Community Problems.* Ed. Cruickshank, Syracuse University Press, 1966.

[2] Denhoff, E. and Holden, R. H., *J. Paediatrics.*, **38**, 452, 1951. Reported in 'Recent Advances in Cerebral Palsy', Ed. Illingworth, 1958, p. 119.

Three of the 36 mothers included in Table 8.III had sought more than one kind of private help. Many of the others had made a single contact and in the 'other' column a variety of contacts contribute to the total—for example, a privately purchased hearing-aid, 'absent' faith healing, a blessing once a year at Lourdes without the child being present. Only 9 mothers had made private arrangements for consultations with specialists. One had done so, without informing the paediatrician in charge of the child, because she felt she needed completely frank discussion of the prognosis and she had not been offered this by the specialist seen for routine care under the National Health Service. There was a strong suggestion from other mothers, too, that in paying for a private consultation one is buying the doctor's time and the right to insist that he spends some of this in giving explanations.

There was little evidence from the East Midlands mothers, then, of extensive 'shopping around'[1] for miracle cures. It was unusual, when other help had been sought, for the mothers to mention it to the paediatrician in charge of the case. The experience of 2 of the 9 mothers who had consulted specialists, or specialist units, privately may go some way to dispel the idea, which seems to be generally accepted whenever this topic is discussed, that to seek further help for a handicapped child is always capricious and unjustified, or symptomatic of an undesirable parental response to the situation.

Mother No. 1 has a mildly handicapped boy of 8; when her son tried to walk at 18 months, he fell frequently. His hands trembled. He was referred by the general practitioner to hospital, where the mother was told there was nothing really wrong. He would improve with time and patience. He did not improve. Father then decided it would be worthwhile to pay for a second

[1] We thought that 'shopping around' might be a peculiarly American phenomenon related to the fact that in the United States of America medical care is still a commodity, to be selected and purchased like any other. Two of the references are American. However, a recently published study of the rearing of handicapped children in America also states, 'The often discussed "diagnostic shopping expeditions" which are inferred to be a characteristic of parents of handicapped children were of minimal incidence in these groups.' Five groups had been studied, one of them consisting of cerebral palsied children. In this last group, 80% of mothers had looked for no opinion beyond that of the first consultant to whom they had been referred.

Barsch, Ray H., *The Parent of the Handicapped Child*. Charles C. Thomas. Springfield, Illinois, 1968.

opinion, and saw a consultant recommended by the general practitioner. A diagnosis of muscular dystrophy was made and the parents told there was no hope of a cure. They were not prepared to believe this and contacted a London hospital, where a diagnosis of cerebral palsy was made after several weeks of investigation with the boy as an in-patient. He was by this time over 3 years old. He began to have physiotherapy and still does. He goes to an ordinary day-school (mornings only), has been assessed by the Spastics Society and will soon go to boarding school. Who knows what the outcome would have been if the parents had accepted either the original consultant's opinion or the second—their first attempt at 'shopping around'?

Mother No. 2 has a severely handicapped boy of 7 years. He cannot walk and his sight and hearing are affected. His speech is impaired. He was referred to a consultant at around 18 months, because he was not walking and could only just sit up. The consultant saw him regularly but said he was just 'slow'—the mother was told by the family doctor that he would never be any better, but he did not say what was the matter. After this, the boy was taken to Lourdes for the first time. The mother later found out from another source that the boy had cerebral palsy.[1] A second trip to Lourdes was made and treated as a holiday for the whole family. He has physiotherapy but has also been treated privately by an osteopath. The mother's main pre-occupation now is to get some kind of education or training for this boy. She provides a very varied life for him, but feels he needs to spend far more time with children his own age. At the time of interview, he was attending a voluntary society day-centre for two days per week. When he was assessed in London, she was told he was not fit to go to school, but she feels that he was upset by the strange surroundings and he would be more likely to perform better if tested in his own home. She may be right. Meanwhile, she too, has some justification for mistrusting expert opinion—her early experience at the hands of the medical profession has not inspired confidence in her, and the consultant told her *that he would take no more interest in the boy if he went to London for assessment.*

This last point is an interesting one—some of the mothers

---

[1] The family doctor had explained to the mother that the child was permanently handicapped but gave no name to the condition. She first found out that he was cerebral palsied when she received a letter from the Spastics Society.

who had not sought a second opinion, suggested that it was possible to offend the consultant in charge if he found out that one wanted to do so, or had done so privately without his permission. They were not willing to take this risk. In other instances, cost was the inhibiting factor. The majority, however, did not seem ever to have entertained the idea of private consultations or treatment. Some had thought about faith healing but had never had an opportunity to contact a faith healer. Yet others spoke of faith healing with a kind of superstitious awe, as something not to be meddled with, particularly if it could really be expected to work. One mother had given it serious consideration but had not, in the end, seen a faith healer because failure might undermine the child's religious faith.

For a variety of reasons, then, the parents of the East Midlands children were, for the most part, not anxious to 'shop around' for medical help nor were they seeking 'miracle cures'. Some of them had been referred to a second consultant by the consultant in charge, but this is not the same as seeking private help on their own initiative. Forty-four (24%) had been referred to one other consultant—an orthopaedic surgeon, for example, or an ophthalmologist—and had seen him at regular intervals. Six (3%) had seen 2 or more such specialists.

Finally, we turn to the question of 'looking ahead' for the handicapped child. This question is intimately related to that of the necessity for permanent residential care, and we expected to find a large proportion of mothers of the severely handicapped children expressing the deepest concern and misgivings about the problem 'who will look after him if/when anything happens to me?' The majority of mothers had seemed to be realistic about the possible need for their children to go away from home at some time (see Chapter 6), and their other ideas about what might happen to their children in the future were equally realistic. Only two mothers gave replies that seemed to us to be unrealistic, because of the youth of the children—one that her 4-year-old wanted to be a doctor, the other that her 3-year-old, whose hands were affected, might be a draughtsman. Three other mothers expressed hopes that medical research might somehow find a way to 'cure' their children but they did not appear to have any real confidence that this would actually happen, and meanwhile said, as did more than half of the whole sample (97, or 54%), that they simply faced each day as it came. Eight of the mothers who 'lived from day to day' in this way expected—and, indeed, hoped—that their children would be cared for in hospitals in the comparatively near future. For others, it was simply accepted as the inevitable long-term prospect. Mothers' comments on this topic ranged from that of the first mother quoted below, who said she could not bear to face the future, to the total resignation of the second mother, whose many troubles had eventually exhausted her capacity for worrying.

Boy: 2 yrs.

I face each day as it comes and just hope that by the time he comes to manhood he'll be able to lead a normal life. I just hope that. I don't think about it a lot because I soon dissolve into tears. I get ever so upset just thinking about it, that I don't think.

Boy: 5 yrs.

Well, I've got so much trouble, like, and nobody to share it with me, that I've got so hard now that I really don't seem to have any more feelings left. I have the feeling that if somebody come in now and said to me that I was—that someone was killed belonging to me at the bottom of the street, I don't know that it would make me feel any worse. I can't explain that kind of a feeling I have, it's just that I've got so hardened against things that I just don't seem to care any more. I don't mean that I'm vindictive to the children or, you know, that kind of a—that part of it at all, it's just that it doesn't hurt any more, d'you know what I mean? And then, it might be God's way of helping me. Of course, I cried myself sick over everything that happened, you know, so that I couldn't eat, I couldn't sleep until I was at the point of getting a nervous breakdown, but now, I mean, I seem to live from one day to another. I don't think about the future and what it brings me, I don't think of what the past has brought me. I just live from one day to the next. At one time I worried about his future, I said to myself 'What will be happening—when I can't be here—what will happen?' but with getting so much worry about money and about different other things, I'm not worried about him as much at all as I should be, as a mother should, I'd say. I don't mean to say that I'm indifferent to him, you know, that sort of a feeling that I don't want him or that—on the contrary, I wouldn't leave him go, but—I don't seem to *worry* about his future any more, you know? I begin to look at—to say to myself, in a few years it'll be all over for all of us, you know, we're not here for ever, you see, that's the way I think now—I don't worry over it any more. It's a good way to be, really.

Some of these mothers pointed out that it was impossible to look ahead at all since no one could tell them how their children would develop. A further 22 of them (12%) simply hoped to achieve very short-term goals for their children, hoping that they would walk before long, or get a place in a school or day-centre. Eighteen mothers (16%) gave answers which showed how they were torn between their desire to plan ahead, and their need to push their inevitable fears and worries about the future to the back of their minds. Only 16 (9%) tried to plan as far ahead as adulthood for their children. In some instances, this had meant taking out insurance policies in the form of endowments, so that there would at least be some extra money available if it should be needed. Others were thinking in terms of buying small businesses where the child could be in 'sheltered' employment. A few of these did not plan in any way but simply felt quite confident that the child was so lightly handicapped that all the normal possibilities would be open to him. Mothers' own words best describe the range of their thoughts and feelings. The examples given below illustrate the kinds of replies that suggested the categorization given in the text above.

Facing each day as it comes

Boy: 6 yrs.

I face each day as it comes. If I try and look into the future—in the future I think Matthew will be happy in a home, and as long as I know he's happy, that's the main thing. I think that's the only thing.

Boy: 7 yrs.

No, I face each day as it comes. I think that was our trouble—we planned ahead what we was going to do, and then *this* came! And so now I don't plan anything . . .

Boy: 6 yrs.

I don't think it's wise to look ahead. You don't know what's going to happen so why worry about it. I never think about it. You just carry on, you know. It's foolish to plan. You don't know what your own life's going to do, never mind thinking about and worrying about the future.

Boy: 7 yrs.

Well, I live from day to day, I do. I mean, I always say, go out and enjoy yourself, you might be dead tomorrow, that's what I always say. If—say—I'd got company come and I'd got washing machine out, I wouldn't say 'I've got washing to do'—bung it back, and that's it.

Girl: 8 yrs.

Dr —— (paediatrician) when she was smaller, one time did say to me, 'Don't look forward and don't look backwards—take each day as it comes' and I've found that's about the best thing to do.

Uncertainty about how the child will develop (included in 54%)

Boy: 3 yrs.

I can't do for one reason—I don't know what's the matter with him. That's how I feel about it. I don't know when he'll walk, or *if* he'll walk, will he walk properly—as we don't know what's the matter with him, no more than Dr —— he can't tell us what's the matter with him.

Girl: 2 yrs.

Well, er, we do kind of think and—you wonder is she ever *going* to be able to walk properly, is she ever going to be able to talk—you talk to various people and I was talking to a lady the other day and she said 'Oh yes, I had a friend and she had a little girl,' she said, 'She sounded something like what Judith is and she said she didn't talk until she was 5 and, but she said she's all right now, she—she's grown up now and she talks but she said she's talked more slowly than you or I would.' She can talk and she is all right and I think that, er, I would like to think that Judith will grow up and will be able to do a job, you see—I think, er, it must be—to have a child and, um, grow up and, um, not be employable, er, must be very difficult. Say to have them at home with you all day long because, um, it must be at the back of your mind, er, what's going to happen to them when we die, you see, for to have somebody like that; but you feel that if they are independent enough to be able to hold a job down, um, then at least they can do that much for themselves but I suppose even so you wonder who's going to, kind of, be in charge of them—when anything happens to you.

Boy: 5 yrs.

Well, I'm beginning just to face each day as it comes, because there doesn't seem to be much you can do about his future, not until you can get him into a training school or something like that. But I've been told there's no hopes until he's seven. So, I mean, it's no good thinking about his future till he's . . . (Who told you that?) Oh, I think it was Mr —— (Mental Welfare Officer). I did ask him about (Junior training centre)—going to school there, but he said they don't take them there until they're 7. But I mean I've never had any offers of, sort of, any other school at all. I know there is other schools but of course they're further afield. No sort of day school—there's only D—— around here where he could go, sort of, daily. And the others are so far away, he'd have to stop there. But I wouldn't mind him going to a training school, definitely, if I could get him in one, because, I mean, then he'd be home for holidays.

Trying not to look ahead but wondering about the future (10%)
Boy: 7 yrs.

Well, I think, as regards to Derek, I think that it's best to face each day as it comes, but I do think about the future. Er—I've often thought of, well, say, what I could do. I mean, I don't know what sort of progress Derek is going to make yet, it's too early to anticipate what sort of progress he's going to make, but I often think about the future as regards to what he could do, if he couldn't be trained for any job of any sort; because you see there is all these places that the Spastic Society are building now for training them in jobs, no matter what type of spastic they are, and even at the training centre where Derek goes, I mean, there's boys there of—well— I mean, twenty that they do find them jobs that would be monotonous ιο us, such as putting in ticket pins and things like that, all in squares of 100, you see, and then pouring them into an envelope. Well, that would be monotonous, but it keeps their mind occupied, and then of course there is—they do rugmaking and things like that. But as regards Derek's future, we've often thought of—I mean, with us having a little bit of land, of what I could do—of something to keep him occupied, you know, probably keeping rabbits or poultry—someting in that line. And if you do have any ideas like that, the Society will always help you with a grant—yes, because I've read of places in the Spastic News. Because I think that's very helpful, the Spastic News. You sort of learn things, you learn of other people's handicaps, of other people—er—other people's achievements, of what they did, and it can give you ideas of what you might come up against. I think it gives you heart. I think it makes you think, well, I mustn't give up, they haven't given up, and they've achieved something, and there's no reason why you shouldn't achieve something with your child.

Boy: 8 yrs.

You look ahead and then you draw away from it a bit. It's no use worrying about something that may never happen.

Girl: 7 yrs.

Well, sometimes I wonder what things are going to be like for her, when she does get sort of in her teens. What jobs will she be able to do? And will she be able to hold a job down? Will she be able to get married? I think she will—there's people in worse conditions than her get married. But the immediate thing is from day to day, I think, coping with it from day to day.

There remains the group of 21 mothers (12%) who fully expressed their fears and worries about their children's future. They had not been able to dismiss these or push them to the back of the mind. These were not exclusively mothers with severely mentally and physically handicapped children. Two of them had children without serious physical or mental handicaps. Their worries were of a different kind from those with seriously handicapped children but were nevertheless real, and concerned the possibility of their children being able to work, after suitable training, and lead independent lives. The other children had severe physical or mental handicaps, or both. Their comments speak for themselves.

Boy: 8 yrs.

That's my biggest worry, as I say, it's worrying about the future. You know, in another 10 years' time, I mean, the way time's going—it's just flown—and the next 10 years are going to go just as fast—well, I'm getting older, and so is he, and the way he's going he'll be massive by the time he's 18 or 19, and . . .

Boy: 8 yrs.

Looking into the future, I only look at the black side and wonder what will happen when we're gone—what happens if we both get killed, or what.

Girl: 7 yrs.

As time goes on and she is still at home, I don't know quite how we're going to cope. Well, for instance, the toilet—I mean, the time *will* come when it will be a bit awkward for (her father) and I don't know how I'm going to cope with her. She's ever so big. But still, we'll come to that when the time comes . . . What would happen if anything happened to either of us?

Boy: 4 yrs.

It would be nice, I think, if he could go just before us, so that we knew he wasn't in the hands of anybody that could possibly hurt him in any way. It worries me—what happens to him afterwards. I wouldn't like to leave this earth and leave him in an institution. He wouldn't be used to that way of life. They're like cabbages in an institution and he's an individual here. He wouldn't understand that. None of my family nor my husband's family could cope if anything happened to us.

One other mother expressed a view very like that in the last quotation given, but with more force, as follows:

Well, I often wonder what *will* happen, because we won't always be here. That (charitable organization) that we're taking him to now— if anything happened to us they would take him into a village and live with all the others who are like him, you see. But if he can't go there and I thought anything was going to happen to me, I'm afraid I'd do something. I wouldn't leave him.

We did not raise these questions with the mothers ourselves. These views were given spontaneously. We do not know how many more mothers had similar thoughts, but it could well be that the few who voiced them spoke for others who had not allowed themselves to acknowledge or express them.

The same may be true of the quotations with which we end this chapter. These mothers express, with courage and honesty, some thoughts which may come to many other parents of very severely handicapped children. Again, these comments were not replies to specific questions on the subject, and are not given here so that a general view may be represented. They are given so that the feelings of individual parents who are living through a tragic experience, may be better understood by all of us.

We often say, 'I wonder what's in store for him'. With all these new drugs coming out, they keep them alive, don't they? You know, I don't agree with it. I don't. I think they should have all these children put to sleep, I do, personally. I said that right from the very start—when you know the children are like this. There should be a law, too. I mean, they're nothing but a handicap to everyone, I think, and my husband as well. As I say, they ought to have done it in the early life. (Interviewer: Sometimes they don't find out till they're older). Well, with (our child) they *did* know what he was going to be like and he's turned out exactly the same as what they told me. The sister at the hospital, she knew, and she didn't believe much and thought they ought to leave him alone. I mean, he would have died if they'd left him alone, you see. We all know that years ago there wouldn't have been a chance and we all said they ought to have left him alone and let him have gone. But there you are. Doctors say they have to save a life, and they did. There's nothing you can do about it.

I think one thing—it's against my upbringing, it's against my religion, it's against everything I want ever to believe and that's one thing I think—I think that with all the aids and with all the help that's given to them, I think myself that they should put them to sleep. It would be more merciful for the child and for the parents to be told the child was dead and never thought of—forgot. Because—it would ruin no bond, really—you know—up to 12 months. Sure, what if you're heartbroken for a while, it's going to wear away, you know? Whereas the ache of this never wears away. That never wears away. Whether I send him away or keep him at home, it's going to be a heartbreak either way, isn't it, you know? I won't feel very happy about it, whereas if he'd been taken as a baby I'd have forgotten now.

CHAPTER 9

THE IMPACT OF HANDICAP—
SOME FINAL COMMENTS

*There are no psycho-social problems unique to the
cerebral palsied.*
*The meaning of cerebral palsy to each patient and each
family is as unique as is personality and life experience.*

GRACE E. WHITE[1]

The two statements which head this chapter (both taken from a
discussion of the social worker's role in relation to handicapped
individuals and their families) may at first sight appear to be
contradictory. However, they express two important points that
we have tried to make in reporting the results of our survey.

There is evidence from other reports and studies[2] that no
specific kind of handicap brings unique problems to the family.
Far more difficulties are shared by all families with a handicapped child than are specific to the medical category of the
handicap.

We have also seen that the East Midlands families meet the
day-to-day problems that handicap creates with patterns of
behaviour that in many respects deviate little from the norms
derived from studying the families of normal children. They
have more similarities with ordinary families than differences
from them.

Having said this, we must stress that we do not therefore imply

[1] White, Grace E. 'Social Casework' in *Cerebral Palsy—its Individual and
Community Problems*. Ed. Cruickshank, W. M. Syracuse University Press, 1966.
[2] See: Barsh, R. H., op. cit.
      Carnegie United Kingdom Trust Report: *Handicapped Children and
        their Families*, 1964.
      Report of the Annual Conference of the National Association for
        Mental Health: *The Whole Truth*, 1964.
      Hare *et al.*, op. cit.
      Tizard, J., op. cit.

that there are no problems attendant upon handicap. Their existence is undeniable and the whole of this study has been an attempt to demonstrate in human terms their real meaning to the people most affected. The struggle to lead the kind of life that seems, to the family concerned, to be desirable and normal must entail varying degrees of effort. Some mothers—often, but not exclusively, those where the child is very slightly handicapped—give the impression that they have had little difficulty in maintaining a very matter of fact attitude towards the child and the total situation. Others show very clearly that they have had to summon physical and emotional resources that they had not known they possessed, in order to meet the challenge of severe handicap. In some circumstances, the mother may find that these resources are already stretched to limit, and the advent of a handicapped child is the final straw. Cerebral palsy, for example, appears to be distributed randomly throughout the population, so that a child with this condition is as likely as any normal child to be born into a family where relationships are not very stable, or where economic circumstances or ill-health of the parents threaten the well-being of its members. The stresses in a family with problems of this kind must inevitably be increased by the advent of a handicapped child, possibly to an intolerable degree.

Even in a family without obvious problems of this kind, the handicapped child will present his parents with a situation which is quite outside their ordinary hopes and expectations. The knowledge that her child is permanently handicapped, that he may never fulfill such hopes and expectations, may arouse in the mother strong feelings for which she is unprepared and does not know how to deal with. Mothers of normal children can share this experience to a certain extent. They, too, are often surprised and shocked when they discover that it is possible, even for the most loving of them, to have hostile and aggressive feelings towards their young children at times. When there is something seriously wrong with the child, other feelings may be added to those that a mother may normally experience— disappointment, for example, or fear that she will not know how to give the handicapped baby the special care that he needs. In some circumstances, mothers may feel resentful that they have been singled out by fate to suffer this catastrophe or, worse still, that they have somehow brought it upon themselves.

One mother in this sample who (like many mothers in the 'normal child' sample in Nottingham) had tried to end an unwanted pregnancy by taking some 'tablets' was haunted by this fear until she summoned the courage to mention it to her doctor, who was able to reassure her. In contrast to this, another mother said that the fact that it was *not* her fault, because she had not done this kind of thing but had wanted the baby very much, made it seem the more 'unfair' that he should be handicapped. These feelings may not always be experienced, many mothers may not experience them at all and for those that do, they may be stronger at one time than at another. Physical tiredness, for example, or family stresses that have nothing to do with the handicapped child, can intensify them.

It is in this context of her own feelings and her own family circumstances that the mother's response to the fact that she has a handicapped child must be unique. However typical her situation may appear to be to an onlooker—a doctor, perhaps, or social worker with wide experience of handicapping conditions—to her it is a completely novel experience. She may know no other mothers in similar situations with whom to compare notes and, like the mother we mentioned in the introduction, she may wonder, not only whether she is caring for her child as others do, but even whether her feelings are shared by anyone else at all.

The replies to our question, 'What is it about (your child) you find hardest to cope with?' illustrated some aspects of this individuality. Just over one third of the replies were so different from one another that they could not be grouped in categories.[1] Similarly, when we asked whether mothers could offer any advice to other mothers of handicapped children, either practical advice on management problems or on learning to face and come to terms with the situation, we found that mothers were reluctant to give answers to the first part of the question. Instead, they either stressed the individuality of each child and his problems or gave very general descriptions of the attitudes they thought it best to adopt.

In the quotations which follow, both the mothers who feel that children are highly individual and those who feel they do not know enough about other handicapped children, are represented.

[1] See Chapter 3.

Boy: 7 yrs.

Each child has individual needs and it's only you that can realize what they are. Everything depends on the actual handicap of your own particular child. If a child is mobile, you haven't got the handicap of the child who's always in a chair. It's difficult to say how your problem fits in with anyone else's because all the children are so different.

Boy: 8 yrs.

I think that is something that grows as the children grow older— you can't give advice on how to cope with the children because each person is different and although you say 'Well, I do this, I'm sure you'd find it beneficial', each child is different. There are no two alike. I can honestly say I don't believe in giving people advice.

Boy: 2 yrs.

Oh, you just have to do what you think's right for him. You've got to think for yourself what's best for him. I don't know anyone who's got any spastic children or anybody with a deaf child like him—nobody—never come across anyone, so I don't know what they do.

Boy: 6 yrs.

No, I don't think so—they've never got owt (anything) the same, have they? Well, I try to help the lady across the road, but she won't let hers go away. I've tried to tell her not to be so silly, like . . .

The mother who speaks next had gone out of her way to meet other mothers, particularly of mentally handicapped children, and felt that she had been able to help them, but not in any specific, describable way.

Boy: 5 yrs.

Well, I've visited a lot of parents with handicapped children and I've made a lot of friends. I find out when they've had a baby mentally handicapped, and I've gone and helped them. And they've all said I've helped them but I can't sort of say anything special— only that it upsets me to see parents that won't take (them out). I had a friend that had a mongol baby and from her finding out, she was *months* before she would take that child out. She wouldn't take her out, off the yard, she wouldn't take her to the shops because of people looking at her. Well, that's silly, because people get to know your children . . . and I think even if they look—er— funny, like—you know—I still think you should take them out.

The next two mothers make the same point about taking their children out and facing the public, but in somewhat different ways. What they have to say may help those who feel the same as the third mother, who follows them and describes her feelings about this very problem.

Boy: 7 yrs.

I think the most important thing for the mother's happiness is to know that people—oh, I should think 99% of the general public—have sympathy and are kind. That you don't have to hide them away and all that, but that most people want to help you. They're curious but they're not nasty.

Boy: 8 yrs.

My only suggestion is—I mean, I don't know whether I'm going about things the right way—but don't spoil them and use your own common sense quite a lot. Be guided by what you think is right for your own child. My only other advice to mothers is—don't give up hope. Take every bit of treatment they'll give your child and that sort of thing, if you know it's what's right for them, and don't be afraid to admit that they're handicapped. I think that *is* a lot of the trouble in lots of cases—people won't admit to having these children and it does seem a shame, you know, because it isn't something to be ashamed of. Actually, I'm very proud of (my child) because he's a very plucky child and he's done well.

Girl: 3 yrs. (*pilot study*)

I'm now finding—of course, I think I've got a bit sensitive—when we go out with her in the pram, people *look* at her now, because she's getting older, you see. We went out with a friend a little while ago and we went in just to have a cup of tea in the afternoon, and she sat on my lap quite well and she had a biscuit, but the waitress said—oh, something like 'Has she got a cold—she keeps very still'. And then two young men came in and made a commotion and she started crying and going stiff. And all those little things seem to get quite big.

And then we went to —— and my husband had to see somebody, so I said 'Oh, well, we'll go shopping.' And I found so many of the little shops were self-service and you can't take a pram in. And there she was, all stiff in the push-chair and I couldn't do any shopping and I came back thoroughly depressed. My husband said 'Oh, what's wrong with you?'—and it seems so, sort of, *feeble*, doesn't it? I know she'd make a to-do at the moment, if I went in and left her (i.e. outside the shops) so I don't. I don't know whether I ought to sort of just tell her and let her yell, but I don't seem as though I can do that. And so I'm afraid I don't go.

This last mother was doubly unfortunate in that she lived in a village in a sparsely populated rural area and had few opportunities to meet other mothers with handicapped children, or to keep up her former interests—she had to walk two miles to get to the nearest library, for example, since having her little girl, whereas before that she could go on her bicycle. She took magazines (*Spastics News* and *Spastics Quarterly*) in an attempt to keep in touch and to be well-informed but found these publications a mixed blessing. What she has to say on this subject is given, along with similar comments, later in this chapter.

Some examples follow of the sorts of attitudes mothers have found it rewarding to adopt towards the task of bringing up their handicapped children.

Girl: 8 yrs. (*pilot study: very slight handicap*)

Perseverance, that's all that's needed, I think.

Boy: 7 yrs. (*pilot study: main problem mental handicap*)

I think, if they can, get them to a school, even if it's only a day school. That does give the mother a break, doesn't it? And get them used to other people as well as be entirely dependent on you. Because I think they can get that way, really.

Boy: 6 yrs. (*pilot study*)

To battle on, to make up your own mind, your own way and keep bashing on along it, regardless of outside 'well-meaners'. I think perhaps one can sometimes feel it's the end of the world, when one needn't at all.

Girl: 4 yrs.

I think myself they need all the love of a normal person—don't leave them out on their own and not talk to them. The like of her doesn't talk but she knows what's going on all around her, just the same, you know. I think myself it's love, really, that they do need. If you leave her for a long time, the like of her that knows everything and can't say anything, they feel left out, somehow.

Boy: 7 yrs.

Only—just treat them as another child. I think that's the best thing.

We turn now to the second half of our question—how would mothers advise others to learn to face handicap and come to terms with it. The whole problem of what is meant by acceptance is raised here.

Whether parents have 'accepted' their child's handicap is a judgment which is scattered through the case histories of families such as these and it is readily apparent both here and in the literature on handicap that the word carries moralistic overtones. The temptation to think of 'acceptance' with approval and 'non-acceptance' with disapproval seems almost irresistible. Moreover, the word is commonly used without explanation or reservation; yet the 'acceptance' of a child's handicap must involve at least two major adjustments on the part of the parents, even before we consider the question (relevant to *any* parents and therefore not to be discussed here) as to whether the child himself is accepted or rejected as a person. The first adjustment consists in the realization of the *fact* of handicap, the acceptance that the diagnosis applies to one's own child. We have seen that the word of the label—'spastic', 'cerebral palsy' or whatever it may be—bears enormous significance in itself for the mother, in the sense perhaps that it gives a form to previously unformed fears; yet it may be that to face the label squarely is necessary before the parents can begin to cope constructively with the problems. Now comes the second adjustment: the decision as to whether one accepts the limitations in the child's development, suggested by a fairly pessimistic diagnostic view, or whether one continually sets one's sights on a developmental standard rather beyond what is to be expected. These are two kinds of acceptance: to make them the basis of a judgment on parental attitudes seems presumptuous, but we can attempt to explore the feelings which lie behind them.

First, we have to try to understand how monstrous the idea that her baby is not normal seems to the mother. No mother ever hopes for a handicapped child in preference to a normal one—such a suggestion is absurd and we all know it. Yet, when ti happens she is expected not only to accept this fact with a minimum of fuss, but also to adjust her behaviour to her child in such a way that she makes realistic allowances for his differences, and, at the same time, treats him like a normal child as much as possible. One mother, who knew very soon after the baby's birth that something was wrong with him, described very well both her feelings at this time and different aspects of her experiences that helped to re-inforce those feelings:

I think any mother, after having a child, goes through a depression period. I felt really depressed and I felt—sort of—the odd one out —not having my baby with me . . . I suppose they've got to be callous and hard to an extent, they can't afford to be too sympathetic towards you but—they sort of *take over* your child, you know. *You* mustn't worry—take things as they come and live day by day, sort of thing. I think you could do with a lot more explaining done to you, really. (Interviewer: Do you think they were 'callous and hard', the way they told you?) Looking back, they probably *weren't*, but to my way of thinking it seemed that way. You probably feel so hurt, especially at that time, that anything anybody said at that time would seem a bit that way inclined . . . When you're told from the very start, *it spoils all the thrill of becoming a mother*, because you're so worried . . . I sort of felt that—rightly or wrongly—I got a feeling it was my fault, which obviously it wasn't, but I suppose some mothers feel that at the back of their minds. . . . I felt differently when I had (the next baby) and he was born normally. I think I felt at last I wasn't one of the outsiders, you know—sort of pushed to one side. At last I'd got a child like everyone else's and I felt much happier towards things.

Most of the mothers in this sample had come to a gradual realization that there was something wrong with their babies, over a period of several months. However, these mothers, too, eventually had to face the fact that this 'something' could not be cured but would affect the child all his life. This realization probably has to be complete before the mother can take the next step, that is, adjusting her expectations of the child and her handling of him to the realities of his disability.

We have discussed elsewhere in this book[1] the parents' dilemma in certain child-rearing situations, where the effort to 'treat the child as normal' has to be realistically related to the extent to which he is capable of behaving (and re-acting to their behaviour) like an unhandicapped child. The attitudes and actions of the parents are vital in this respect, because it is largely through them that the child begins to learn how to regard himself. He in his turn will have to learn how to capitalize

[1] See Chapter 4.

on his capabilities and at the same time to accept his limitations. The parents, and later the child himself, must walk a tight-rope between acceptance of the fact that he is different from other children and insistence that he should be like them in as many ways as possible. If they emphasize his differences, continually 'make allowances' for his disability and learn a habit of helping and shielding, they may be branded 'over-protective'; if they minimize his handicap, treat him as an ordinary member of the family and speak with optimism of his mental attainments or physical prospects, they may be judged to have 'failed' (sic) to accept the situation.

How the balance is to be maintained is a problem that, in the end, has to be solved by the individuals concerned. There are strong pressures by society upon the handicapped 'to deny their disabilities and impel them to strive to be non-disabled. We do not wish the disabled to 'accept' their disability. On the contrary, we insist that they deny it.'[1] This pressure is expressed, for good or ill, in a number of ways—in the attempt to accommodate handicapped children, wherever possible, in ordinary schools; in the exhortation to mothers by medical and other advisers, to 'treat him like a normal child'; in the emphasis placed on the achievement of independence by the handicapped and the encouragement they receive to take their place in the 'normal' world of work and of social interaction. The ambivalence of society only becomes apparent when the disabled want to be treated as having normal adult needs, desires and sensitivities and find that these are not recognized. Handicapped people often complain, for example, that casual social contacts tend to address their contacts rather than themselves—'Does he take sugar in his tea?' Marriages between the handicapped, particularly if the couple want to have children, commonly provoke adverse comment. Disabled adults often find it difficult to find jobs in the field of their choice; they are expected to work if possible but only in those areas which the normal world considers appropriate and in which it is prepared to make adjustments to accommodate them. Briefly, the handicapped person's world is often circumscribed to a degree far greater than his disability dictates and this he is supposed to accept.

[1] Meyerson, Lee. *Somatopsychology of Physical Disability*. In: 'Psychology of Exceptional Children and Youth.' Ed. Cruickshank, W. M. Staples Press, London, 1956.

Given considerations such as these we have outlined here, it seems by no means obvious that 'acceptance' is either a good or a bad attitude in any general or absolute sense. Should a mother accept a 'hopeless' prognosis for her child, for instance, and consequently give up striving for him? An interesting auto-biographical account of a mother who refused to do this is given in *One of Those Children*,[1] which tells of Mrs Neal's total commitment to helping her cerebral palsied child to develop. She achieved remarkable success, in spite of the lack of support from medical and other advisers. Perhaps the rest of her family suffered—perhaps the rewards were small in proportion to the effort. Is it for others to make judgments of such a mother? The problem is hers, and the decision on how best to meet it must be hers too.

The determination not to give up but to fight for one's child against a too-ready dismissal of his developmental potential, in the face of the contradictory attitudes that we have suggested can exist, and against the more obvious failures of society to make suitable practical provision for him, has been demonstrated more than once in this book. 'There's only one way to get anywhere . . . and that's to bang on the table'—'—having to fight all the time for the child, which you *do* have to do'—'To battle on.' The mother who speaks next felt that to be able to fight, to go on believing and hoping that things would improve for her child, was an important aspect of her being able to tolerate the situation.

Boy: 8 yrs.

Well, I think you've got to keep fighting, you've got something to fight for all the time. *Yes, I think once you lose that bit of a hold, everything's gone.* You're always hoping that something will turn up, that something's going to be there. There again, it's no good moaning about it, it's there and you've got to do it, haven't you? That's what gets me so annoyed with these people—'*I* couldn't do it'. I mean, you've *got* to do it. That's one of the silliest things. I think it depends on you—what type of person you are. If you're going to manage, you'll manage.

The concepts of acceptance and adjustment share the difficulties that surround those of guilt, over-protection and over-dependence which we have discussed elsewhere in this book:[2]

---

[1] Neal, Elizabeth. *One of Those Children*. Allen & Unwin, London, 1961.
[2] See Chapter 4.

they describe complex patterns of feeling, attitude and circumstance in terms so grossly over-simplified as to distort almost out of recognition the original response (part emotional, part rational, part expedient) of the individual parent. Possibly as an immediate consequence of this simplification, such concepts all too easily lend themselves to woolly theorizing; conveniently amorphous, they can be shaped to fit anyone's favourite prejudice. Invariably the parents seem to be the losers, in the sense of submitting oneself to the value-judgments of others and losing one's individual voice under a blanket generalization.

Because we feel unable to justify any categorization of parents in these terms, we have not attempted to analyse statistically their 'acceptance' of the situation in which they find themselves, and which brought them into this study. In the last resort, too, there are considerations of courtesy which must restrain us from 'intruding, uninvited, into the privacy of another's mind and feelings',[1] let alone evaluating such feelings against ill-founded hypotheses. It is our function here, to listen to what mothers want to tell us, and to offer their comments to others in the hope that they will be accepted in the spirit of helpfulness which prompted the mothers to talk to us in the first place.

There are, however, certain features which some replies have in common. The parents of the least handicapped, for example, tended to feel that there was little for them to accept, like the father speaking in the next quotation.

Boy: 5 yrs.

He's never been handicapped as far as we're concerned, because he's never been that trouble, to *be* handicapped. I mean, he does exactly as the others do. If he only does it with one hand, he still does it. And he never complains about it.

Some mothers emphasized the point that, once faced with the fact of having a handicapped child, they had no choice *but* to accept it.

Girl: 7 yrs.

Well, I suppose you *do* come to terms with it. Nobody'll do anything about it *for* you.

---

[1] Sheridan, Dr Mary, op. cit.

Boy: 7 yrs.

Well, all I can say is, have patience. To help them a bit, but not a lot—you know—to be able to do things for themselves. And to love them. That's all. Well, you've just got to accept it, I mean, if they're handicapped, you can't do anything about it, can you?

Girl: 7 yrs.

Well, this is it, isn't it? You have got to face it. I mean, it's reality in itself. You can't just dismiss it from your mind. It's there, so the best thing I can say is, face up to it. Do the best you can for the child and face it. It's there and it's going to stay with you.

Boy: 7 yrs.

Well, you've just got to learn to live with it, haven't you? I mean, you've got it—you've got the child and you've just got it to bring up and got to learn to live with it—it's surprising what you *do* do!

Others described how difficult it had been to accept the facts at first.

Girl: 6 yrs.

I think if you accept that they are as they are, that's half the battle. I mean, if you can't accept that your life's a misery; *mine* was, till I got used to the idea that she was as she was and nothing on earth will alter her. If they can do that and have another child—if they've only got one, definitely to have another child. That's helped me a lot, really.

Boy: 8 yrs.

We were more or less a month or two before we could really make ourselves believe it was true. We just thought they'd made a mistake, which I think you do. And until you've learned to accept it, I don't think you can get anywhere. You can't do anything because all your mind does is go around—'Where can we take him that they'll tell us they've made a mistake?' You can't cope with it that way, you've got to accept it first.

Boy: 5 yrs.

Well, the only thing I've found is just to accept it and not fight against it. I think at the beginning I did sort of try and fight against the thought that he was a spastic but I've come to the conclusion that it's no good fighting against it, that it's there and there's nothing else you can do about it. They said 'Do the best you can for him and hope for the best.'

Boy: 2 yrs.

Well, if a mother feels like I did when I first had Jeremy—you know—I was willing to *give* him away, because of him being like (that). I think it's because when you think of a handicapped child you think of its handicap all over the body. It's not going to be any use to you or the baby (itself).

Boy: 8 yrs.

Mind you, it's not nice at first when you're told but you get over that, sort of overcome it, you know, you get over that stage. Mind you, I used to sit and cry hours, I did, because he could only sort of creep, drag himself across the floor.

The opposite point of view was also expressed. These mothers did not gradually learn to accept the handicap after refusing to face it in their young babies. They found that it was to some extent more acceptable when the children were young but that they could not face the implication that the children would continue to be handicapped when they grew older. This was most often expressed when mothers referred to books, magazines and to meetings of the Spastics Society local groups. Some found radio and television programmes upsetting for the same reason.

Boy: 7 yrs.

The first thing I did was go to the library and (the bookshop) to see what I could find, and the only book that I could get was a book on educating spastics which was very good. And I've lost it, someone I lent it to hasn't returned it to me. I'm sorry I haven't got it, because actually it would be more use to me now than when I bought it, when he was a baby. Because I read half of it and thought 'This isn't going to apply to me.' You don't realize that your child's going to be as handicapped and you don't face up to it, you *won't* see it . . . I went through a period when I didn't want to go (to meetings of the local group of the Spastics Society) mostly because I didn't want to see the older people, the older spastics. I think you go through a phase when you think, 'My child will never be like that.'

Girl: 3 yrs. (pilot study)

I must confess those magazines depress me terribly. I've only got to see the various people or children in them and—you can't but wonder if your own child will be like that.

We end this chapter—and this book—with the words of the mother of a severely mentally and physically handicapped child of six.

> You've just got to accept them for what they are and not keep wishing they were something else, not keep wishing they were normal. Well, you naturally *wish* they were normal, but it's no good to keep longing for them to do things that you know they can't do. You've just got to accept them for what they can do.

'You naturally *wish* they were normal.' This mother surely speaks not only for the mothers who contributed to this survey but for all mothers of handicapped children. She expresses precisely their first and final dilemma—the acceptance of the unacceptable.

APPENDIX I

The Spastics Society is a voluntary body which exists in order to promote the welfare of cerebral palsied children and adults. It has a central organization consisting of an Executive Committee, the paid officers of that committee and a small number of members. The headquarters of the Society are in London. The main body of the Society consists of the members of the Local Groups, the majority of which are affiliated to the central organization of the Society. It is important to remember that every Local Group is an independent body, with its own constitution, its own committees, its own fund-raising schemes and its own range of services. These vary according to the needs that are given priority by the group in any one district. A list of Local Groups and their services is published by the Society in 'The Spastics Society Year Book 1968', which is obtainable through the Society.

This pamphlet also lists the many services, including schools, hostels, assessment services, publications and advisory services of all kinds which are administered by the central organization.

The relationship between the central organization and the Local Groups is maintained in a number of ways and is the special responsibility of the Society's Regional Officers. One such officer is based on each of the 6 regions into which England and Wales have been divided for this purpose. His function is to act as a liaison officer with the London headquarters and as co-ordinator of local effort. He acts in an advisory capacity to the Local Groups in his region.

Any-one wishing to contact the Society can do so either through the secretary of the Local Group or the Regional Officer. The latter will be listed in the telephone directory under 'Spastics Society'. If there is no telephone number listed for the Local Group secretary, his or her address can probably be obtained from other sources—the Regional Officer, the Council of Social Service or the Citizen's Advice Bureau for example. Alternatively, direct contact can be made with the London headquarters of the Society at this address:

> The Spastics Society,
> 12 Park Crescent,
> London W.1.

APPENDIX II

Glossary of terms commonly used in discussions of cerebral palsy.

This list is taken from the Spastics Society handbook *The Early Years*.

Abduction   Movement of a limb outward and away from the body
—i.e. raising an arm or a leg out to one side.

Acalculia   Inability to do the most simple calculations.

Achilles Tendon   The 'heelcord'; the long tendon which joins the
calf muscles to the heel. It can easily be felt at the back of the
heel.

Adduction   The opposite of 'abduction'—i.e. movement of a limb
towards, or even across, the midline of the body.

Aetiology   The study of what is known of the cause of a disease.

Agnosia   Inability to recognize objects or sounds due to lack of
perceptual capacity, although the general level of intelligence is
normal.
   (a) *auditory agnosia,* where the person's hearing is normal but
   he is unable to understand what words mean.
   (b) *finger agnosia* (sometimes used as a test for cerebral palsy),
   where a person is unable to identify individual fingers when,
   for example, they are touched by another person.
   (c) *tactile agnosia,* where a person is unable to identify familiar
   objects by touch alone although he is aware that he is
   touching something.
   (d) *visual agnosia,* where a person is able to see but unable to
   identify objects visually.

Aphasia   A specific defect of brain function which leads to:
   (a) *expressive aphasia,* when a person is unable to express ideas
   in words.
   (b) *receptive aphasia,* when a person is unable to understand
   spoken language.
   Auditory agnosia and receptive aphasia mean much the
   same thing.

Apraxia   An inability to perform purposeful movements, such as
using a screw-driver, which is not accompanied by any apparent
muscular weakness. It is due to a dysfunction of the brain.

Ataxia   A generalized inco-ordination of movement due to inco-
ordination of the muscles involved which results in instability of
sitting, standing and walking and a similar disturbance of arm
movement.

Athetosis   The term used to indicate a particular sort of movement and posture which prevents or seriously impairs normal movement and result from a particular brain lesion. It is presented in the 'athetoid' type of cerebral palsy.

Atonic Diminished resistance to passive movement of the segments of the limbs of the patient.

Audiogram A record, in the form of a graph, of the hearing acuity of a patient.

Audiometer, an instrument used to test a patient's hearing acuity at different frequency levels and intensity.

Cerebellum That part of the brain which—among other things—has to do with balance.

Cerebral palsy 'A disorder of movement and posture arising in the early years of life as the result of some interference with the ordinary development of the brain.' It is non-progressive in that the damage to the brain itself will not get worse, although the symptoms may change from time to time.

Diplegia Paresis (weakness) of the upper and lower limbs of both sides. Diplegia is usually understood to imply that the lower limbs are more severely affected than the upper (of double hemiplegia).

Distractibility The inability to concentrate—i.e. a person who is easily distracted from the performance of a task.

Double hemiplegia Paresis involving the limbs on both sides of the body with the upper limbs more severely affected than the lower.

Dysarthria Imperfect production of the sounds used in speech due to defective neuro-muscular control of the organs which control speech.

Dysgraphia Difficulty in writing due to a defect of brain function other than sensory defect. (The alternative word 'agraphia' is sometimes used.)

Dyslalia Difficulty in speaking due to a defect of brain function other than sensory defect. (The alternative word 'alalia' is sometimes used.)

Dyslexia Difficulty in reading due to a defect of brain function other than sensory defect. (The alternative word 'alexia' is sometimes used.)

E.S.N. (*Educationally sub-normal*). A person whose intellectual ability is such that he is unlikely to benefit fully from education in an ordinary school and who may do better in a special school more suited to his abilities.

Emotional disorder A loose term used to indicate abnormal behaviour and emotional disturbance. This disorder is not due to a psychosis (q.v.) but to some emotional strain or stress.

Epilepsy A condition which causes a person to suffer from fits characterized by abnormal and uncontrollable movements. Such fits are described as 'grand mal' when there is loss of consciousness and convulsions or 'petit mal' when there is only momentary loss of consciousness and no convulsions.

Equinus See *Talipes.*

Extensor The name given to those muscles which, when they contract, cause a joint to straighten.

Flexor The name given to those muscles which, when they contract, cause a joint to bend (or flex).

Gastrocnemius muscle The bulk of the muscles at the back of the calf.

Grand mal See *Epilepsy.*

Hamstrings A group of three muscles at the back of the thigh which extend the thigh at the hip and flex the leg at the knee.

Hemiplegia Weakness or paralysis of the limbs on one side of the body as the result of a disorder of the brain.

Hyperkinesis Incessant restless activity.

I.Q. (Intelligence quotient) A figure used to indicate the level of a person's intelligence above or below that of an 'average intellect' (I.Q. 100). Intelligence Quotients are based on responses to Intelligence Tests (q.v.). Education, mood, drive, energy, sensory receptors and perception play a part in determining the use a person makes of his intellectual capacities.

Intelligence Test A test used to measure a person's intelligence. Numerous tests have been devised to give a numerical indication or I.Q. (q.v.) of a person's intellectual capacity. Although no ideally satisfactory tests have so far been designed, experienced psychologists, using groups of tests, can make a useful estimate of a person's intelligence.

Kinaesthesia The sense and understanding of where one's limbs are, whether still or in motion.

Monoplegia Paresis or paralysis affecting one limb only.

Ophthalmologist A doctor who specializes in diseases of the eye.

Paediatrician A doctor who specializes in the care of children and their disorders and diseases.

Paralysis, paresis, palsy These words are often used rather loosely. Strictly speaking, 'paralysis' means complete inability to move a particular part of the body. 'Paresis' describes a weakness not amounting to paralysis and 'palsy' is synonomous with paralysis. In fact, many people use 'paralysis' to describe weakness only.

Paraplegia Weakness or paralysis affecting the legs only.

Perception A process of the brain by which we understand and interpret the information we receive through the organs of sensation, which keeps us in contact with the outside world by means of vision, hearing, touch, smell and taste.

Preservation   A persisting tendency to repeat actions, phrases or sentences.

An inability to stop one activity and transfer to another.

Petit mal   See Epilepsy.

Psychiatrist   A doctor who is concerned with mental disorders. A child psychiatrist specializes in the mental and emotional disturbances of children.

Psychologist   A person who studies the ways in which people think and act. He is usually the person who assesses intelligence and applies intelligence tests.

Psychosis   A mental illness, other than intellectual handicap (subnormality) in which the patient does not have insight (i.e. does not understand that his mind is not working normally). A psychosis is a more severe and fundamental 'illness' than a neurosis.

Quadriplegia   Weakness or paralysis affecting all four limbs. See also tetraplegia.

Reflex   A stereotyped automatic movement without conscious control—i.e. sudden withdrawal of the hand when pricked with a pin or the jerk of the lower leg when the knee is tapped by the doctor.

Retarded   A word used to indicate development—physical or intellectual—which is less than average for a person of the same age. Often used to indicate suspected mental subnormality, or as a euphemism for 'mentally subnormal'.

Rigidity   Sustained stiffness of a limb or limbs in extension.

Sensory   Having to do with that part of the nervous system which *receives* and interprets signals through the senses as distinct from 'motor' which has to do with that part of the nervous system which *transmits* signals to the muscles and so organizes the activities of the body.

Spastic   A term with two meanings:
  (i) Popularly used to indicate any child or adult suffering from cerebral palsy.
  (ii) Medically speaking it is used to describe a specific type of stiffness commonly seen in the limbs in hemiplegia and diplegia. This is detected by the particular sort of increased resistance to passive movement of the parts of the limb.

Spatial perception   The appreciation of size, distance and the relationship of objects one with another.

Talipes   The medical word for clubfoot. A deformity of the foot in which the foot is pointing downwards (equinus) or upwards (calcaneus); pointing downwards and turning inwards (equinovarus) or pointing downwards and turning outwards (equinovalgus); drawn upwards and turned inwards (calceneo varus) or drawn upwards and turned outwards (calceneovalgus).

Tetraplegia Weakness or paralysis affecting all four limbs. See also 'quadriplegia'.

Tonic Sustained tension in a limb.

Tremor Rhythmic, uncontrolled repetitive movements of parts of the body.

Triplegia Weakness or paralysis affecting three limbs.

Valgus, Varus Terms used to describe the position of a limb distal to the joint under consideration. If the part beyond the joint points away from the midline, there is said to be a 'valgus' joint. If it points towards the midline the joint is said to be varus.

ERRATA

Appendix II, page 212

'Preservation' should read 'Perseveration'

The Family and the Handicapped Child

UNIVERSITY OF NOTTINGHAM
CHILD DEVELOPMENT RESEARCH UNIT

City/County ....
Interviewer ....
Date.................

GUIDED INTERVIEW SCHEDULE
(For mothers of C.P. children, aged 1–7 years)

BACKGROUND

Child's full name..

Present at interview?...........

Address...

Date of birth.................... *Sex:* Boy/Girl
Family size and position (for each child in family, indicate sex and age; include foster children, marked F and deceased children marked D. Mark respondent *)

sex

age

N.B. Note here whether any siblings have physical or mental handicaps or chronic ill health.

MOTHER: Age.... *Not working/working part-time/full-time*

Former occupation ....

Occupation if at work.....................
Did you train for a job before you had children? *(details)*

FATHER: Age.... *Precise occupation*...............
Does he have to be away from home at all, except just during the day?
Home every night/up to 2 nights away p.w./3 nights + p.w./

normally away/separation or divorced/dead/other..............

Shift work? YES/NO *What shifts?* ....

Does any other adult live here now, apart from your husband and yourself?

YES......................................./NO

If YES: How does N get along with him/them?

MOVEMENT

1. Does N have much difficulty in moving or   *Score*
   controlling his limbs? *(underline which)*   No   0

		slightly	*badly*
If YES which limbs are affected?	*Rt. leg*	1	2
	Lt. leg	1	2
	Rt. arm	1	2
	Lt. arm	1	2

2. Can he walk at all?

   (N.B. If child seen to be walking, ask: What help does he need with walking?)

   Details:

Independently	0
With some *support*	1
With much *support*	2
Person *needed throughout*	3
No	4
Under 2 years old	0

   If walking at all: When did he start walking as well as this?

   ....

   If M. reports balance only *affected, note this*...............

3. *If* walking *at all, ask:* How far can he walk like this?

Completely mobile	0
To local shop or school	1
Around house and *up and down the stairs*	2
Enough to get around the house	3
Two or three steps only	4
Not walking	5

4. Can he move in any other way, crawling for example, or shuffling or wriggling along the floor? *Yes (specify how)*

   ....

Around house and up and down the stairs	1
Around house (not stairs)	2
Around one room	3
No	4
N/A	0

   If NOT walking

5. If he's lying down, can he get up into a sitting position alone or do you have to help him?   *Alone*   0
                                                   Helped   1

6. Can he stay sitting up without support, on the floor or in bed?

YES	0
NO: *Hard chair* without *arms*	1
Hard chair with *arms*	2
Needs to be secured in chair	3
Only in special chair or pillow arrangement	4

How long has he been able to sit like this?..................

7. Can he get on to his feet without help?

YES	0
With support (e.g. furniture)	1
With help from person	2
No	3

How long can he stand like this? *As long as he likes* 0
2–3 mins. (e.g. for dressing or toilet) 1
Few seconds only 2
Not standing 3

How long has he been able to stand as well as this?
If NOT walking, crawling, sitting, standing:

8. Is there *any* way he can move himself without help? NO 1
(i.e. voluntary total *body movement,* not *falling forward in chair involuntarily or similar* involuntary *movements)*
Prompt if necessary (i) Can he roll over when he's on the floor? YES 0
(Details)
(ii) Does he have any difficulty in holding his head up?
YES 1
NO 0

EQUIPMENT

9. Does he have a wheelchair? NO/YES *Self-propelling*
Not self-propelling
Collapsible
Not collapsible

Do you have any other special equipment for N. such as:
Amesbury chair
Frame-walker—wheels
Frame-walker—legs
Baby 'bouncer'
Special Seat/baby-relax/babysitter
Toilet seat
Other (specify)

Ask 'Is it bought or lent?' *for each*
If lent Who is lending it to you?

10. *If any equipment:*
    Have you found the.....................a lot of help to N?
    RATING: Total functional mobility: How far can N go un-accompanied, with equipment if applicable?

11. And has it been helpful to you or do you find it difficult to handle in any way?

12. Did you have a lot of trouble getting it/them?
    How long was it between the time it was ordered and the time you got it?

13. Is there anything you've asked for but haven't got?

14. *If any borrowed equipment:*
    Who suggested to you that you could borrow this equipment?

15. Have you got a car?   YES/NO
    If YES: Does N have special straps or seat in it?   YES/NO
    Does he need someone in the car to hold him?
    (apart from the driver)   YES/NO
    Will the wheel-chair fit into it easily?   YES/NO

16. How far can N do other things for himself?—can he put on any of his clothes without help?   YES/NO
    Which? ....
    Can he manage buttons zip-fasteners shoes, boots, slippers
    YES/NO   YES/NO   YES/NO
    Can he *take off* any of his clothes?
    Which? ....
    N.B. *Note whether clothes worn are normal for age. If N not present, ask*
    Do you find the usual sorts of clothes convenient for N?
    YES/NO
    If NO, ask: What special clothes does he wear?

FEEDING

17. We'd like to know something about N's mealtimes now. Is he a good eater or do you have any trouble about that?
    good/varies/finicky
    If finicky: What do you do about that?
    battles/persuasion/permissive/anxious

18. Does N have any difficulty in chewing or swallowing ordinary food?

No	*0*
Yes, but eats ordinary food	*1*
Yes, can take minced or mashed foods only	*2*
Yes, can take liquids and purées only	*3*
Yes, still completely bottle fed	*4*
TOTAL:	

19. Can he feed himself or does he have to be fed?

Feeds himself	0
Can feed himself but so slow and/or messy, M. feeds him	1
Has to be fed	2
Under 2 years old	0

Can he drink from an ordinary cup?   YES/NO
Can he hold an ordinary cup?   YES/NO
Does he ever use a feeding bottle?   YES/NO
Can he use an ordinary spoon?   YES/NO
   Total feeding handicap, Q.15–16

20. And does N have his meals with the rest of the family or do you find it easier to give him his meals on his own?

CONTINENCE

21. How much help does N need when he goes to the toilet?

Unaided	0
Under 4 years old	0

Describe (analyse difficulty)
Does he have trouble over moving his bowels?
If YES: Do you do anything about that?

22. Can he tell you when he needs to go to the toilet? *(by any method, including pointing, special cry, etc. Note which.)*

Bowels:
Under 2 years old 0
Yes 0
Sometimes 1
No 2

Bladder:
Under 2 years old 0
Yes 0
Sometimes 1
No 2

23. I expect he still wets his bed occasionally, doesn't he?   *Yes* 1
   No 0

How often?   *Under 3 years old* 0
Does he still have accidents sometimes in the daytime—wetting his pants?   *Yes* 1
   No 0
   Under 2 years old 0

If not got, prompt:
Do you know what the main reason is—does he have trouble actually *controlling* his bladder, or is it just that he doesn't get there quickly enough?
   Yes 1
Does he dirty his pants at all?   *No* 0
   Under 3 years old 0

If any accidents: What do you do when he wets his pants? What do you say to him?
   punitive/rewarding/disapproving/supportive

24. *(If appropriate)* Do you use nappies for him during the day?   YES/NO

If YES: Have you been supplied with any
                   nappies?
                   Who by?

25. And does N have any fits or convulsions or 'bad turns' of any
    kind?

If *YES:* How often?	*No*	0
What are they like?	*Isolated*	1
How long do they last?	*Monthly*	2
Do they come at any special time of day?	*Weekly*	3
What seems to start them off?	*Daily*	4

          Mostly severe/occasionally/severe/never severe/none

26. What about his general health—is he often ill, apart from his
    handicap?
    NO/YES ....

If not mentioned: trouble with teeth	YES/NO
bronchial trouble	YES/NO
urinary infections	YES/NO

    Prompt: Has he had any illness in the past?

SPECIAL SENSES

   Sight

27. Has N had any trouble with his eyesight?

	Normal	0
	Don't know	0
	Repaired squint	1
	Impaired (no glasses)	1
	Squint	1
	Glasses	1
	Blind	2
	TOTAL:	

   Hearing

28. Or with his hearing?

	Normal	0
	Don't know	0
	Impaired (no hearing aid)	1
	Hearing aid	1
	Severely deaf	2

APPLIANCES

29. Does N wear special boots or shoes/calipers/*other (specify)*
    .... /*none.*
    If YES: Where do you take him to have his...............
    fitted?
       (include glasses or hearing aid if applicable)

How often do you have to go?
Who do you get in touch with when they need to be mended or altered?
Have you had any trouble in getting them?
Or in getting them repaired?
(If not mentioned, prompt): Do you find this very expensive?

SPEECH

31. *Either*   Has N started to talk yet?

Normal for age	0
1 or 2 words only	3

Or *if N obviously talking:* How much does
N talk now?

Slight difficulty	13
(e.g. impaired but can be understood by all	
Speech defect but can be understood	2
after short acquaintance	
Great difficulty	3

If YES: When did he start to
talk (as well as this)?   *(only M/family can understand)*

Unintelligible	4
No speech	5
Mute (because deaf)	5

* *Interviewer's rating of active vocabulary,*
   to be made at end of interview:

Apparently normal	0
Poor	1
Negligible	2

32. Does he seem to understand what *you* say to him?

   everything/most/a little/nothing

   If under 4 years
   If you say to him 'Where's the pussy, baby, tick-tock, Daddy'—
   or any other appropriate thing—what does he do?
   If over 4 years and appropriate
   Can he give a simple message for you? (e.g. can he tell his Daddy dinner's ready)?

33. *If appropriate*
   Does he take a lot of interest in what's going
   on around him?

Normal	0
Some interest	1
Completely apathetic	2

34. Does he understand he mustn't touch things like the fire and gas-taps and electric points?

35. Can you tell me any little way N has thought of for himself to make it easier for him to dress/eat/reach things/tell you what he wants/other
   Describe:

36. *If over 5 years:* Can N read or write at all yet?
    If NO: Does he know any of his letters?

* *RATING*

   Child clearly of 'normal' or above average intelligence/uncertain/
   confirmed defect

37. Has he been tested by the educational
    psychologist?   *YES/NO/Don't know*
    If YES: Where was that done?
         Home/hospital/school/London/ ....
         (by whom) Education/Health/Spastics Soc./ ....
    How old was he then?
    Do you know what the result was?

38. Does N go to a school or to a day-centre, or does he have a
    home-teacher?
         No/ordinary school/special school/day-centre/home-teacher
         If home-teacher, state hours per week:

39. *If NO:* Would you like him to go to school/day-centre or have
    home-teaching? YES/NO Any special reasons?

40. *If YES to school or centre:* Where is that?
    How does he get there?   How long does it take?
    How often does he go?   And for how long each time?

41. *If YES to any of 34:* Do you find this helpful to N?
    In what ways?

42. And is it helpful to you? *(Probe:* Do you find you are able to
    carry on the training he gets yourself?)
    Can you go to the school and talk to them about N whenever
    you like?
    Have you done that?

CHILD'S CONTACT WITH FATHER (from 4-year-old schedule)

43. How much does your husband have to do with N? Does he:
    Bath him? O/S/N   Dress him or undress him? O/S/N
    Read to him *or* show him a
       picture book?   O/S/N
    Tell him stories or sing to
       him?   O/S/N
    Help him with exercises?   Resp./S/N/no exercises
    Take him out without you? O/S/N
    Look after him while you're
       out?   O/S/N
    If NEVER to any of these: Is that because he doesn't want to or
    because you don't want him to?

44. Is there anything else your husband does for N?............
   ....O/S/N
   Is there anything he won't do—that he draws the line at?
45. Does your husband look after the other children a lot?

* *RATING*
(Father with N)	*Highly/fairly/non-participant*
(Father with sibs)	*Highly/fairly/non-participant*
(M. re F. & N)	*Very satisfied/dissatisfied/not shown*
(M. re F. & sibs)	*Very satisfied/dissatisfied/not shown*

46. Have you or your husband (or anyone else) been able to make any gadgets or equipment for N yourselves?   NO/YES
   Details
   Is there any gadget you would like to see made that you can't make yourselves?

47. Has your husband made any alterations to your home for N?
   NO/YES

   Details
   Is there anything about the house you find inconvenient?
   (Prompt if necessary: Are there any awkward steps or doorways?)
   Can you move the wheel-chair around the house?
   Has the local council helped you in any way—by widening doorways, or fitting rails or ramps, or in any other way?
   NO/YES

   Describe:

48. *Check-list of housing amenities:*

Toilet:	Bath:	Hot water
Inside	*No*	*Yes*
Outside	*Yes, shared*	*No*
Not flush	*Yes, not shared*	*Connected to bath*
Upstairs	*Upstairs*	Garden:
Downstairs	*Downstairs*	*Accessible for N*
Same floor	*Convenient for N*	*Inaccessible but N*
Shared	*Inconvenient for N*	*put there*
Convenient for N	*Not used for N*	*Not used*
Inconvenient for N		*None*
Potty normally used		Yard:
		Accessible for N
Washing Machine? YES/NO		*Inaccessible but N*
		put there
Drying facilities		*Not used*
No problem/problem..............		*None*
Number of living rooms:		

49. Where does N spend most of his time during the day—*in his pram/cot/chair/playing on the floor/in the {garden/in the house/ at school/other/* .... {*yard*
    (*Check room where most time is spent if this is not mentioned*)
    Does he sleep at all during the day?
50. Where does he sleep at night?
    Do you have any trouble getting him to sleep?   YES/NO
    If YES: How do you cope with this?
    Ask ALL: Does he have a dummy or anything else to cuddle or suck at night?   NO/YES...............................
    (*If sedatives not mentioned, ask:* Does he have any tablets or medicine at bedtime? Does he have any tablets or medicine during the day?)
51. Does he sleep well once you have got him to sleep?   YES/NO
    Who usually gets up in the night when he wakes?
    What do you do to get him back to sleep?
    Does he disturb any other members of the family? (*Specify*)

CONTACTS WITH OTHER PEOPLE

52. Some people say that having a handicapped child makes a mother very lonely.
    Do you think this is true, from your experience?
53. Do you go out visiting at all?
    Do you take N with you?
    Do people come to see you?
54. How does N get on with people outside the family?
55. Is he ever upset by them?
56. Do you find that your friends and neighbours are helpful?
57. (*Unless already got*) Do you see much of your relatives?
    Have they been a help to you and N?
58. How does N get on with them?
59. Are you friendly with any other mothers of spastic children?
    Relatives: None/isolated/adequate/much support
    Friends: isolated/adequate/much support

CONTACTS WITH SOCIAL SERVICE AGENCIES

60. Now we'd like to know about other sorts of help that you've had with N. Does the Health Visitor from the clinic call on you to see how he is getting on?   YES/NO/NOT NOW
    How often?
61. Has anyone else come to see you about N—from the Spastics Society, for instance, *or the Friends of Spastics/school welfare/ health department/church orgnization/Invalid Children's Aid/ other*
    How often?

62. *If any visits:* How do you feel about these visits? Have you found them helpful?
    If NO visits: Have you asked them not to? YES/NO
    Prompt, if necessary: Did you have any particular reason for not wanting them to call?
63. Could you do with more visiting? (*specify what kind*)
64. What sort of visits do you think could be most helpful—advice about special problems or just a friendly chat?
65. If you wanted help or advice, who would you turn to?
66. Would you say your own doctor has been a lot of help to you? YES/NO
67. Do you belong to the local group of the Spastics Society/Friends of Spastics?
68. *If YES:* How did you hear about the Society?
    How often can you manage to attend meetings?
    If NO: Did you know about these groups? YES/NO
    If KNOWS: But you still didn't want to join. Can you say why?
    If DOESN'T KNOW: Would you have joined if you had known about it?
69. Do you belong to any other group or club? YES/NO *(Details)*
    e.g. W.I./T.G. or a church group or anything like that?

MEDICAL SUPERVISION

70. Does N go for a regular check-up by the doctor? YES/NO
    How often?
71. Does he usually see your own doctor for this or a doctor at the hospital? *G.P./hospital doctor/no regular check-up*
72. Does he always see the same doctor? YES/NO *(Give details)*
73. How do you get there? *Own transport/public transport/private taxi/paid-for taxi............................/hospital transport/other.......................*
74. How long are you usually away from home altogether?
    How long do you have to wait usually?
    And how long do you spend with the doctor?
75. Do you ever find that you have to break appointments? YES/NO
    If YES: What is usually the reason?
76. *If sibs:* Last time you went, who looked after the other children? *Relative..................../neighbour or friend/children at school/children taken/no other young children.*
77. How helpful are these routine visits?
    (Prompt all): Do you think they should be *more frequent/less frequent/longer time spent with doctor/same doctor should see him every time/own doctor should look after N.*

78. *If NOT GOT:* Do you regularly see any other hospital specialist?
    Where is that?
    How often?
79. And how convenient are those visits?
80. Can you think of anything else to do with the hospital(s) that
    might be improved? *(How?)*
81. Apart from his check-ups, does N attend anywhere for treat-
    ment of any kind?
    No/speech therapy/occupational therapy/physiotherapy/other

    ....
    How often?
    And where is that?
82. Do you have to go with him?
    How do you get there? *Own transport/public transport/
    private taxi/paid-for taxi.........................../hospital
    transport/other........................*
    How long does this keep you away from home each time?
    *(If possible, get travelling time..................../waiting
    time.................../treatment time.................)*
83. Does you husband ever take him to hospital or for his treatment
    without you? U/O/S/N
    Does he ever go with you? U/O/S/N
    Husband normally responsible for certain visits (specify)......

    ....
84. Do you find it difficult in any way to keep these appointments?
    YES/NO
    Note reasons:
        e.g. cost/time/awkward journey/care of sibs/other..........
85. If you could choose, how would you improve the arrangements
    for this sort of treatment?
86. Can you think of anything that would make the treatment
    itself more useful to N?
    (Prompt if appropriate: Have you been shown any special ways
    of feeding him, holding him, sitting him up?)
87. Do you carry on with the treatment at home? YES/NO
    If NO: Are you supposed to?   YES/NO
    What is the main difficulty?
    If YES: Do you have any difficulty with that?
88. Some people say that it's worth while getting special treatment
    that you can't get from the hospital. For instance, have you
    ever taken N to an osteopath or bone-setter?
    If YES:
        When was that?
        Where did you see him?

How did you hear about this treatment?
How often did you go?
How long did you keep on going?
Did you pay for this yourselves?
How much did it cost you?
How much good do you think this treatment has done for N?
Does the doctor at the hospital know about it?

89. Have you ever been to a faith-healer about N?   YES/NO
    Details as in Q.88.

90. Have you had any other sorts of treatment or advice from anyone outside the Health Service?   YES/NO
    Details as before:

SEPARATION FROM MOTHER

91. Has N ever been separated from you for more than a few days?
    Has he been to hospital or a residential centre or school at all?
                                                        YES/NO

    Age of child   Where?   Length of stay   Reason

92. *If YES:* Were you able to visit him?   YES/NO
                How often?
    If NO VISITING: Was that because visiting wasn't allowed or was there some other reason? *(Specify)*

93. Would you say that N behaved differently when he came home again—was he upset at all?   *YES/NO/NO SEPARATION*

94. And have *you* ever had to go away from *him*—to hospital or anywhere else?
    Age of child   Length of Separation   Reason
    Did that upset him?

95. Has your own health been fairly good since N was born?
    Do you find that you get very run-down or depressed? YES/NO
    If YES: Is your doctor giving you anything for that?
    If possible specify: sleeping tablets/tranquiliser/tonic/other......
    ....

TIME OF BEING TOLD OF C.P.

96. We are asking all the mothers we talk to how they first came to know that their children might be spastic.
    Can you tell me when *you* were first told that N might be handicapped?
    (How old was he?)
    Who told you?

97. Had you any idea before this that all wasn't well with him?
    YES/NO

98. *If YES:* What made you think that?
Did you tell anyone what you thought? YES..........⁄NO
Prompt: Did you discuss it with your husband?

99. When your doctor/the specialist told you about N, what did he actually say to you?

100. Has either your own doctor of the specialist taken a lot of trouble to explain N's difficulties to you? (For example, has anyone discussed with you what makes it difficult for N to balance/talk/get clean?/—*or as appropriate to the child in question.*)

101. Do you feel you understand his handicap as well as you want to, or would you be glad to have it explained more fully?

102. And how do you feel about the *way* you were told?

103. What do you think is the right moment to be told about these things?
Prompt: Do you think the doctor should tell the parents as soon as he *suspects* something is wrong, or should he wait till he's quite sure?

104. After you knew what was wrong with N, did you try to find out more about handicapped children? For example, did you send for any of the booklets published by the Spastics Society?
                                        YES/NO
Has anyone at the hospital shown you any booklets—the physiotherapist, for example?   YES/NO
Have you read any other books about the subject, or articles in magazines?   YES/NO
Have you heard any talks on the radio? YES/NO
Were they easy to understand?   YES/NO
Were they helpful to you?   YES/NO

105. Has the doctor discussed the question of having more children with you?   YES/NO
Have you discussed this with anyone else? YES........ ⁄NO
(Prompt if necessary: Husband)

106. Do you think having N (has) changed your feelings about having more children in any way?   YES/NO

107. And did you do anything about birth-control? YES.... ⁄NO

MANAGEMENT OF CHILD

108. Well, now, we'd like to know something about how you manage to fit in your housework with looking after N.
Does anyone give you any help with the housework? YES/NO
Who?   How often?

109. What about shopping—do you take him with you? YES/NO/SOMETIMES
If NO: How do you manage your shopping?

110. Do you find that other mothers stop and talk to you about N, and take an interest in him?   YES/NO

111. Some mothers of handicapped children say that's something they don't like. How do *you* feel about it?

112. And do you take him on other outings (with the other children) —to the park, for instance?
Any other places?

113. About how long can you leave him in a room on his own while you get on with other things?
(State whether N is left in pram/cot/chair/on the floor/other . . . .
. . . . .)

114. And how long will he amuse himself *(if helpless)* be peaceful and happy without wanting your attention?
(a) while M. is in sight (or hearing if N is blind)
(b) while M. is not in sight (or hearing if N is blind)

115. What does he like doing best—what is his favourite occupation?

116. What toys seem to give him most pleasure?

117. Do you keep any pets?   NO/YES . . . .
Is N particularly fond of the. . . . .?

118. If you could buy anything you liked for his next present, what would you choose?

119. Is N a happy child, or is he miserable a lot of the time?

120. Does he want a lot of cuddling?   YES/NO
Do you manage to give him much time on your lap?   YES/NO
And how about his Daddy—does he cuddle N?   YES/NO

121. Is he easy to manage or does he object to having things done for him?

122. Does he ever have a real temper tantrum?   YES/NO
If YES: How often?   What starts them off?
            What does he do?   How do you deal with it?

123. *If N is mobile:*
Would you say that N gets in as much mischief as most children of this age?
What kinds of mischief?
If appropriate: Do you think he does these things on purpose?

124. What sort of things seem to upset or worry N?
How do you cope with this? (Do you try to avoid upsetting him as much as posible, or do you find it easier to let him get upset and calm him down afterwards?)

DISCIPLINE (from 4-year-old schedule)

125. Children of this age often don't want to do as they're told. What do you do when that happens with N? *(Discount danger-ous situations)*

If sibs: Do you do this with the other children too, or do you find that you have to try to manage N differently from them?

126. If he refuses to do something he really must do, what happens then? *(If M. says 'I make him', prompt:* How?)

127. Do you ever promise him a reward for being good?   YES/NO
(Prompt: What sort of goodness would that be for?)

128. How do you feel about smacking? Do you think it's necessary to smack most children?   YES/NO
And N?
(Would you feel the same if N were not handicapped?)

129. Do you smack N *simply* as a punishment or do you have to be really angry or at the end of your tether?

130. What sort of naughtiness do you usually smack him for?

131. Do you think smacking does him any good? (*Prompt*: In what way?)

* *RATING:* A. *Smacks only when calm/only in anger/both/ almost never*
  B. *M. believes in smacking/disapproves in principle*
  C. *Excludes N because of handicap/makes no differ- ence between N and others/no sibs.*

132. Is there anything else you do when he's naughty?

133. Do you ever send him to bed or put him in a room by himself as a punishment?   YES/NO

134. Do you ever say he can't have something he likes—sweets or television, or something like that? (as a punishment)   YES/NO

135. Do you ever tell him you won't love him if he behaves like that?   YES/NO

136. *OMIT IF CHILD IS ATTENDING*
Do you ever say that you'll send him away, or that you'll have to go away from him if he's naughty?   OMITTED/YES/NO

137. Do you ever threaten him with somebody else—his Daddy (or his teacher or the doctor—someone like that?)   YES/NO

138. *If M. says NO to any of these (133–7).* Would you do any of these things if N were not handicapped?   YES/NO

139. *(If child is 3+ and talks):*
Do you think it's important for him to say he's sorry when he's done something wrong? Do you ever make him do that, even though he doesn't want to?
Makes/No/Speech inadequate

140. *If other sibs:* Do you think you make allowances for N more than for the other children?   YES/NO
Do they understand that this can't be helped or do they think he gets away with things and that this isn't fair?

141. Do the other children ever seem jealous of N for the attention he gets?
   I think where there's a handicapped child the other children often *do* feel a bit left out. What do you do about this problem?
142. Do you have much trouble over the other children's behaviour generally?
143. On the whole, are you happy about the way you handle N's behaviour or do you sometimes find yourself doing things you don't really approve of?
144. Do you agree with your husband about this or is he a lot more strict or less strict than you are?
145. Do you and your husband always agree about how N should be brought up generally, or do you feel differently about some things?

LEISURE ACTIVITIES

146. Have you had a holiday since N was born?   YES/NO
   If YES: Did your husband⎫   YES/NO
            N   ⎬ go too?   YES/NO
            the other children⎭   YES/NO
   If N taken with family/parents: Did you find your accommodation yourself?   YES/NO ....
   If N not taken: Who did you leave N with?
   If NO HOLIDAY: If you could have found suitable accommodation to take N to, would you have gone?
   If you could have left N in good hands for a few days, would you have gone without him?
147. Would you let him go to a residential centre so that you could have a break?
148. Has N ever been on holiday with other handicapped children? YES/NO
   If NO: Has this been offered to you?   YES/NO
   Would you be glad for him to do this?   YES/NO/LATER ON
149. Suppose you had to go away unexpectedly—into hospital or something like that—what arrangements would you make for N?
   And for the other children?

BABY-SITTING (from 4-year-old schedule)

150. Do you and your husband ever manage to leave N/the children so that you can both go out together?
   1 p.w.+/1 per month+/seldom/1 or less p.a.
151. What happens when you do that? (*Prompt:* Does somebody come in? Do you pay her?)

Paid baby-sitter/unpaid/(specify) ....
neighbour listens/other children responsible/nobody resp./......
....

152. Do you ever go out without your husband?   YES/NO
     Does he ever go out without you?   YES/NO
153. Do you ever leave N at someone else's house for a while?
     *Almost daily/2+ per week/1–2 per fortnight/occasionally/never
     (excl. school)*
154. How does he seem if you leave him with somebody else? Does
     he mind you leaving him?   YES/NO
     If YES: What do you do about that?
     If NO: Was there ever a time when he minded?   (age)........
     What did you do?
155. Do you always tell N when you're leaving him, or do you find
     it easiest to slip off without him knowing?
156. *If there are sibs:* Does it make a difference if he is with the other
     children when you leave him?

ATTITUDE OF OTHER SIBS TO N

157. Does/do the other child/children bring their friends home to
     play in the garden/yard or house?
158. *If YES:* Do they take an interest in N? Do they talk to him?
     YES/NO
159. Do the children include N in their games at all?
160. When they go *out* to play, in the street/park, for example, do
     they ever take N with them?
     *O/S/N/sibs too young to take resp./N too handicapped to
     go/*................................
161. Does N ever go out to play in other children's houses or in the
     park/street with other children?
162. What do you do if he gets into a disagreement or a quarrel?
163. In general, do you find it possible to leave N to settle his own
     differences at this age?
164. Suppose N complains to you of another child, what do you do?
165. Does he ever hit another child back?   YES/NO
     Do you encourage him to stick up for himself in this sort of
     way?   YES/NO
     If YES: Can you give me an example of when you might do
     that?
     If NO: Is there any situation in which you might do that?
     YES/NO
     EXAMPLE in either case:
166. Does N do his share of starting quarrels? Does he torment the
     other children?

*RATING: ENCOURAGEMENT OF AGGRESSION IN
SELF-DEFENCE*
　　general encouragement/special circumstances/never
　　Child's actual behaviour: passive/adequate/aggressive

MOTHER'S OPINION OF HANDICAP

167. Talking generally now—what do you feel is N's greatest handicap, from his point of view?

168. And from your point of view—what is it about him that you
find hardest to cope with?

169. Would you allow N to go to a residential school or training
centre or home when he's old enough? Does your husband
agree about this?　YES/NO

170. *If this is projected, note: when for?　age*....................
Where?
Do you think this is the right age for him to go or would you
prefer it to be earlier or later?

171. At the moment, who do you rely on most for help?
(If HUSBAND)—and who after him?

172. Can you think of any kind of help you would like that you
haven't had?

173. Have you any suggestions to make that might be helpful to
other mothers of handicapped children—either practical suggestions for looking after their children, or on how you manage
to face this and come to terms with it?

174. And what about the future—do you ever try to look ahead and
make plans for N, or do you face each day as it comes?
Probe if necessary:
Have you any ideas at all about N's future?
To be completed after interview:
　　Appearance of child:

HOUSING

　　*Modern detached/modern semi/Victorian detached/Victorian
semi/terraced with bays/terraced without bays/self contd. flat
......flr,/rooms......flr./......council house on estate/
council house, not estate/council flat......flr./other........
....
　　D............*

LIST OF REFERENCES

BARSCH, RAY H. *The Parent of the Handicapped Child.* Charles C. Thomas, Springfield, Illinois, 1968.

BICE, H. V. in *Cerebral Palsy—Its Individual and Community Problem* Ed. Cruickshank, W. M., Syracuse Univ. Press, 1966. 'Parent Counselling and Parent Education'.

BOLES, G. *Personality Factors in Mothers of Cerebral Palsied Children.* Genet. Psychol. Monogr., 1959, 59, 159–218.

BOTT, ELIZABETH. *Family and Social Network.* Social Science Paperbacks, London, 1968.

CARNEGIE UNITED KINGDOM TRUST. Report—*Handicapped Children and their Families.* 1964.

DENHOFF, E. and HOLDEN, R. H. *Pediatric Aspects of Cerebral Palsy.* J. Pediatrics 39, 363, 1951.

DENHOFF, E. and ROBINAULT, I. *Cerebral Palsy and Related Disorders.* McGraw Hill, New York and London, 1960.

ELLIS, E. *What the Doctor has to Offer* in Teaching the Cerebral Palsied Child, Ed. James Loring, Spastics Society/Heinemann, London, 1965.

FINNIE, NANCIE R. *Handling the Young Cerebral Palsied Child at Home.* Heinemann Medical Books London, 1968.

HARE *et al. Spina Bifida Cystica and Family Stress.* British Medical Journal, September, 1966.

HASKELL, S. *Some Speculations on the Effects of Sensory Deprivation upon Cerebral Palsied Infants and Adults*, in Learning Problems of the Cerebral Palsied. Report of a Study Group held in Oxford 1964, The Spastics Society.

ILLINGWORTH, R. S. *Recent Advances in Cerebral Palsy.* J. & A. Churchill Ltd., London, 1958.

KELMAN HOWARD R. *The Brain-damaged Child and his Family* in Brain Damage in Children — the Biological and Social Aspects. Ed. Birch Herbert G. Williams and Wilkins, Baltimore, 1964.

KERSHAW, JOHN D. *Handicapped Children.* Heinemann, London, 1966.

MEYERSON, LEE. *Somatopsychology of Physical Disability* in Psychology of Exceptional Children and Youth, Ed. Cruickshank, W. M., Staples Press, London, 1956.

Ministry of Health Annual Report 1966/67. H.M.S.O., 1968.

NEAL, ELIZABETH. *One of Those Children.* Allen & Unwin, London, 1961.

NEILSON, HELLE. *A Psychological Study of Cerebral Palsied Children.* Munksgaard, Copenhagen, 1966.

NEWSON, E. *Provision for the Pre-school Child* in Graduate Women at Work. Ed. Constance E. Arreger.

NEWSON, J. & E. *Infant Care in an Urban Community.* Allen & Unwin, 1963.

NEWSON, J. & E. *Four Years Old in an Urban Community.* Allen & Unwin, 1968.

NEWSON, J. & E. *Child Rearing in Socio-cultural Perspective* in The Spastic School Child and the Outside World. Spastics Society/ Heinemann, London, 1966.

OSWIN, M. *Behaviour Problems Amongst Children with Cerebral Palsy.* John Wright and Sons Ltd., Bristol, 1967.

QUILLIAM, T. A. *Clinical Communication—a Contemporary Problem.* Med. Bio. Illust., 15, 66–68, 1965.

Report of the Committee on Local Authority and Allied Personal Social Services. (The Seebohm Report) Cmmd. 3703, H.M.S.O., London, 1968.

Report of the Annual Conference of the National Association for Mental Health. *The Whole Truth*, 1964.

ROITH, A. I. *The Myth of Parental Attitudes.* The Journal of Mental Subnormality, 9, 51–54, 1963.

SCHAFFER, H. R. *The Too-cohesive Family—A Form of Group Pathology.* The International Journal of Social Psychiatry, Vol. X, No. 4, 1964.

SCHONELL, E. *Educating Spastic Children.* Oliver and Boyd, Edinburgh, 1956.

SHERIDAN, M. *The Handicapped Child and His Home.* National Children's Home, London, 1965.

Statistics of Education, H.M.S.O., 1965 and 1966.

TIZARD, J. *Community Services for the Mentally Handicapped.* O.U.P., London, 1964.

TOWNSEND, P. *The Family Life of Old People.* Routledge and Kegan Paul, London, 1957.

WHITE, GRACE E. *Social Casework* in Cerebral Palsy—Its Individual and Community Problems. Ed. Cruickshank, W. M., Syracuse Univ. Press, 1964.

WIGGLESWORTH, R. Symposium on *The Handicapped Child* in The Practitioner, No. 1150, Vol. 192, April 1964.

WIGGLESWORTH, R. *The Value of Early Part-time Developmental Training* in The Spastic School Child and the Outside World. Ed. James Loring and Anita Mason, Spastics Society/Heinemann, London, 1966.

WILLMOTT, PHYLLIS. *The Consumer's Guide to the Social Services.* Penguin Books (Pelican Original), 1967.

WRIGHT, BEATRICE A. *Physical Disability—a Psychological Approach.* Harper and Row, New York, 1960.

YOUNG AND WILLMOTT. *Family and Kinship in East London.* Routledge and Kegan Paul, London, 1957.

INDEX

SOCIAL SCIENCE LIBRARY

Manor Road Building
Manor Road
Oxford OX1 3UQ
Tel: (2)71093 (enquiries and renewals)
http://www.ssl.ox.ac.uk

This is a **NORMAL LOAN** item.

We will email you a reminder before this item is due.

Please see http://www.ssl.ox.ac.uk/lending.html
for details on:

- loan policies; these are also displayed on the
  notice boards and in our library guide.

- how to check when your books are due back.

- how to renew your books, including information
  on the maximum number of renewals.
  Items may be renewed if not reserved by
  another reader. Items must be renewed before
  the library closes on the due date.

- level of fines; fines are charged on overdue books.

Please note that this item may be recalled during Term.

305334670V